INTERMITTENT FASTING FOR WOMEN OVER 50

The Ultimate Guide for Beginners with Delicious Recipes to Lose Weight Fast, Increase your Energy, Detox your Body and Live your Healthiest Lifestyle

Melissa White

TABLE OF CONTENTS

INTRODUCTION

Intermittent Fasting is essentially the practice of restricting mealtimes, reducing snacking, or cutting out days of eating, based on the method one chooses. So many of us snack unconsciously or when we're getting moody without any real hunger. So many of us eat unconsciously in general, and then we're confused why our bodies are holding onto the weight. Intermittent Fasting reminds the body what food is for, and it restarts that nutritional absorption potential. All you have to do is cut out the snacks, fast a few hours a day, or just drink water a few days a week.

IF is both a dietary choice and a lifestyle, but those who have the most success with IF will tell you that it became a lifestyle for them almost instantly. Sure, dieting plans and IF can match up nicely, but for some, IF requires no dietary change whatsoever. The point is to eat less and to eat less often. The brain and the body will respond in no time.

Fasting, intermittent fasting, in particular, should not be mistaken for a diet, for improving your life is a meal planning schedule. Dieting is not a bad practice, but it is a struggle to fight the desire to eat a certain type of food, so it only diminishes your desire to continue with it while fasting is easier and you can get used to it more quickly as it only conditions your body to new eating habits. Fasting helps your body and mind to know that you don't have to be fed continuously, so you eat less and reduce your digestive system's pressure. It also allows you to stop eating as a result of stress or as a convenience that is not wellbeing or a healthy way to handle difficult situations at all.

It is safer to use the resources that would otherwise be used to digest food and heal the body and wash the system. Physiologically, the body is put in a state of rest, so the body can regenerate, rebuild and reinforce the weakened organs. It also allows the body space through a process called autophagy to rid the cells from waste and stored contaminants.

Nonetheless, you need to limit the practice for that time in order to be effective effectively, otherwise, you will not see any health improvements. You must reduce the levels of stress and practice relaxing practices such as relaxation. Energy conservation for the fasting period should be a big part of your plan.

Before making any major improvements in life that would affect your life, it is always best to contact a health professional.

Hence, making people believe that women do not indulge in intermittent fasting, which we don't agree. If done tastefully, intermittent fasting has resulted in excellent health and weight loss benefits for women. So in this chapter, we will go thru exactly how intermittent fasting effects women in all aspects, such as hormones, hunger craving, and many more things are on the agenda. With that in mind, let's get started.

CHAPTER 1
WHAT IS INTERMITTENT FASTING?

If there was one word that could describe the intermittent fasting, it would be the word, "fasting". What a no-brainer! This is actually correct. Fasting is the gist of this method of eating pattern. It is one of the most popular diets used nowadays. However, it is quite interesting to note that despite being called a diet pattern, intermittent fasting is more about being an eating pattern. There is a huge difference between dieting and intermittent fasting. How?

In most of the dieting patterns, you get to eat specific diets at specific times and schedules. In most of the diets, certain foods are to be taken into some portions and some edibles are to be avoided. That is not the case in terms of intermittent fasting. There is really no restriction on what to eat and what to not consume. The approach of avoiding certain foods can be combined with intermittent fasting for enhanced effectiveness but that is given at the later stage.

One of the best things about intermittent fasting is that it is free of time restrictions. Literally, there is no restriction on this method. You can follow it for two days, a week or a month. Or you can follow it for six months after which it will become a life style. However, one thing that needs to be noted is that for reaping proper benefits of intermittent fasting, you would have to do it for at least a few weeks, preferably a month. Although, the method of intermittent fasting doesn't come with any side effects, it still needs to be done for long time to reap benefits. You can leave this peculiar eating pattern at any time without any harmful effects.

It is interesting to know that some of the motivations behind intermittent fasting are not related to diet at all. Fasting has been present for a very long time. The first and most obvious reason behind fasting is simply religious or spiritual devotion. In religions like Islam, Christianity, Hinduism and Buddhism, the fasting is done for religious purposes. The simple act of fasting is said to increase the spiritual prowess of a person.

There is also the reason of tight schedule which inspires people to take up this style of eating. Some of us have no time for breakfast and intermittent fasting comes as a rescue. One can still follow the style of healthy eating even with the habit of skipping breakfast. Another reason why some people take up the act of intermittent fasting is because of physical fitness and weight loss. This is one of the most popular reasons why this eating pattern is adopted.

Does intermittent fasting work?

An interesting thing to observe is that the intermittent fasting has a lot of supporters along with those who claim it is a useless technique. Why? For die-hard diet fans, the weight loss is not achieved without giving up certain foods. Intermittent fasting places zero restrictions on such diet restrictions, therefore, it doesn't seem effective to some people. However, that is not the case.

Most of the methods of intermittent fast revolve around limiting our meals and snacks to a specific time. The time frame is usually chosen between 8 to 6 hours within a day. In one of the methods, the meals are decided to be taken in any eight hours of a day while the remaining sixteen hours are to go without a food intake. Despite the claim of critics, the intermittent fasting has been proved by science. It provides many benefits including those of health, weight loss and general cholesterol.

So how does it work for weight loss? There are many mechanisms to prove that it does. Science has shown that the act of restricting your meals to a time window does wonders. The best wonder that it does is the reduction of calorie intake. It is a blessing for people who want to reduce their weight.

The calorie intake is quite important for weight loss. Usually, the weight gain is caused when calorie intake is more than calorie consumption. The extra calories are stored as fat. Thus, for weight loss, it is crucial that body functions are consuming the calories properly.

When the meals are restricted to a window of time, this restricts the intake of calories. It is a boost to calorie consumption. How? Suppose you do your breakfast. That will obviously lead to flow of calories in your body. When you plan your next meal within next eight hours, it will be another calorie intake. However, when you don't consume anything for the next sixteen hours, you are letting your body consume the calories that were taken in. Those calories are consumed properly and no extra calories are stored as fats. Your body will adjust to it more and more. It will naturally lead to weight loss. This is just one mechanism of how intermittent fasting works for the weight loss. There is also another advantage of intermittent fasting that actually ends up implementing weight loss effectively. That advantage is the increase in production of a hormone called, "neropinephrine". This is a special hormone that boosts metabolism. When your metabolism is faster, you end up digesting the calories effectively. This is a big boost to the weight loss. Furthermore, there is another benefit of intermittent fasting. It effectively reduces the hormone called insulin. This is often responsible for management of sugar levels in blood. The reduction of this hormone leads to more fat burning than usual. I don't think I need to link this to weight loss since it is quite obvious.

Furthermore, there is another benefit of intermittent fasting. That is the retention of muscle mass. Naturally when calories are consumed properly, not much is added to the fat ratio of body. This will lead to the retention of muscle mass that will naturally lead to better form. It is indirectly related to weight loss if your extra weight was caused by fat. There are many researches which state that your body fat will reduce and weight loss will occur by intermittent fasting.

Personally, I always prefer combining the approach of calorie intake with healthy eating. Some of the foods have more cholesterol than others. Therefore, take care that if your breakfast had a lot of calories, your next meal should be one that balances it out. This will leave plenty of room for your bodily development. Some people reduce the effects of intermittent fasting by consuming only the oily foods with lots of fats. When the weight loss doesn't work like it should, they think the intermittent fasting is not an effective method. If they could only make effective adjustments to their diets, they could reap its benefits much faster. Furthermore, trying out intermittent fasting for a few days or one week and expecting weight loss is like planting a seed and expecting a tree next week. The process works only if you follow it for at least 3-12 weeks. I believe if you commit yourself to first four weeks, it will become an effective lifestyle. You will not be giving up anything. In fact you will be eating without the worry of it adding fat on to you.

There is one thing that I need to be clear about here. The term of weight loss refers to reduction of fats and toning of your body to proper form. The weight loss will rapidly occur if it was caused by fats accumulated in your body. Some people don't measure their progress by weight loss since their bones are naturally heavy. That is perfectly fine. As long as your body is getting slimmer and is gaining proper form, who cares about the weight loss anyways?

The weight loss was added since majority of women above fifty often are overweight. The routine is brilliantly applicable to you even if you are doing a job or you are a housewife. However, intermittent fasting has its effectiveness proven by many other mechanisms.

Seeing the other benefits of intermittent fasting, it is crucial to notice that reduction of insulin doesn't just aid the fat burning process. It is essentially crucial for diabetes which some of the ladies over fifty tend to suffer from. The reduction of insulin is particularly effective for controlling the blood sugar levels. The blood sugar is quite a problem for ladies above fifty and this gives another reason for ladies to give this effective method a chance.

Furthermore, the intermittent fasting is also helpful in reduction of cholesterol. This cholesterol reduction is linked to improving heart conditions. Some of the ladies above fifty suffer from heart diseases and this adds yet another reason why intermittent fasting is effective.

I believe after this, you will be convinced that the intermittent fasting is actually a proved technique for weight reduction and health benefits.

CHAPTER 2
INTERMITTENT FASTING FOR WOMEN OVER 50 INTRODUCTION

A woman's body is a delicate creation! While a man can engage in many stress-inducing activities (such as extended fasting, extreme dieting, and intense workouts) without any significant effects on their body, females aren't designed to handle such high amounts of stressful impact, and for a good reason. The female body is designed to house another human to ensure the continuation of the human race. Whether or not a woman chooses to get pregnant and give birth during her childbearing years, it doesn't change her chemical composition. She is still a woman with very sensitive hormones. What impact does it have on the female hormones, especially for women over 50?

Your Hormones at 50+ Years

One of the major health concerns for women over 50 is menopause. Luckily these major hormonal changes leading to menopause don't just happen overnight, it takes anywhere from 3 to 15 years for these changes to happen, make an impact, and for hormones to become relatively stable. That's a long time to endure these unpleasant feelings. On average, women experience menopause at age 51, but it can occur as early as the 30s in some women and as late as the 60 for others (Stoppler, 2019).

At the onset of menopause, when your chemical messengers are unstable, it is not uncommon to wake up some mornings and feel as if you've just run a marathon on crutches. Your hormones can fluctuate dramatically and cause you to become sensitive like never before The initial symptoms such as hot flashes, night sweats, dry skin, hair loss, tender and small breasts, insomnia, vaginal dryness, low sex drive, and of course, mood swings are indications of perimenopause.

The female sex hormones (estrogen and progesterone) are unstable during this period. In some postmenopausal women, testosterone levels become higher than estrogen and progesterone levels and can result in insulin resistance, higher triglycerides (too much fat in the body that can lead to heart attack, stroke, and heart diseases), and a higher risk of developing breast cancer (Yasui, et al., 2012).

When you've gone a full 12 months without menstruation, most of these early symptoms will subside. Some will even disappear altogether because, at that stage, your hormones have stabilized or are in steady decline. But there's still one major problem: weight gain. It is normal to put on some weight during perimenopause and menopause. A little extra padding can even be beneficial at this stage of life. The fat tissues can be your body's extra if you get sick and as estrogen gets down-regulated by your ovaries, your fatty tissues step in to up-regulate.

However, when your estrogen levels become too high in relation to your progesterone levels, it can result in significant weight gain, especially in the waistline or on the hips. To achieve a healthy weight at this stage of your life, you will need to be deliberate about maintaining the balance between these hormones. Besides the sex hormones estrogen, progesterone, and testosterone, let's briefly look at how other hormones that control your weight (with particular attention on insulin) can be effectively managed.

Insulin Resistance

Weight gain has been linked to insulin resistance in postmenopausal women. Except for the obese, insulin resistance seems to play a role in weight gain for many postmenopausal women, especially those with lower BMI (Howard, et. al, 2004). But what exactly is insulin resistance? What are its causes, and how can you prevent or manage it?

Think of the hormones in your body as command centers that deliver instructions to your cells. The hormone insulin instructs them to extract sugar (glucose) required for body fuel from your blood. In a healthy person, the cells receive this instruction and promptly comply. But when the cells begin to ignore the insulin command center – specifically the cells in the muscles, body fat, and liver – the person is labeled as insulin resistant. Their cells are no longer responding to the instructions from insulin to extract glucose from the blood. This refusal to comply with instructions from the hormone insulin means that your body no longer has unfettered access to its fuel (glucose) and can't function optimally.

Although your body fights courageously to defeat these disobedient or resistant cells by producing more insulin, the battle cannot go on indefinitely. After a while, the cells of your pancreas will grow tired of producing more and more insulin. Soon, your pancreas will throw in the towel. If this happens, it won't be long before excess glucose accumulates in your blood since it is not being extracted and used for fuel. Excess blood sugar levels can result in Non-Alcoholic Fatty Liver Disease (NAFLD) – a precursor to liver damage and heart disease. Also, too much glucose in your blood can increase the risk of developing prediabetes and type 2 diabetes (American Journal of Managed Care, 2013).

Factors such as smoking and being overweight (obesity) can lead to insulin resistance. Other factors include age, excess fat, especially in the belly region, a sedentary lifestyle, and poor sleeping habits, particularly sleep deprivation.

Symptoms of Insulin Resistance

Metabolic syndrome. If at any time, you begin to have any three of the following symptoms, it is a strong indication that your body is resisting naturally produced insulin:

• High triglycerides: Triglycerides are a type of fat found in your blood. When triglycerides levels become equal or greater than 150 mg/dL, it is likely to increase the hardening of the arteries. There is a higher risk of heart attack, stroke, and other heart diseases if that happens.

• High fasting blood sugar: Blood sugar or glucose levels are usually slightly higher in the mornings, that's why it is called fasting blood sugar. Healthy blood sugar levels are usually between 80 – 130 mg/dL before meals and below 180 mg/dL about two hours after eating. But when fasting blood sugar exceeds the normal levels, it could be an indication of a metabolic syndrome.

• High blood sugar: Also known as hyperglycemia, high blood sugar refers to elevated levels of glucose in the blood. It can cause frequent urination, frequent feeling of thirst, and a higher volume of glucose in the urine. Blood sugar level is said to be high when it is above 130 mg/dL before eating or above 180 mg/dL after eating.

• High blood pressure: A blood pressure higher than 130/85 mmHg is indicative of a metabolic syndrome.

• Low high-density lipoprotein levels (HDLs): HDL cholesterol, also called the good cholesterol, helps your body to get rid of other forms of harmful cholesterol from your system. An ideal HDL level is 60 mg/dL and above. A level less than 40 mg/dL is not healthy.

Excess fat on your waistline. If your waist area is beginning to show signs of accumulated fat, it might be an indication that you are developing insulin resistance. And if unexplainable dark patches begin to show up on your skin, particularly behind your neck, groin, or armpit, it could be an indicator. Usually, this only occurs in severe cases of insulin resistance and is known as acanthosis nigricans.

Preventive Measures

The good news is that it is possible to prevent and even reverse insulin resistance, especially at its onset. As a woman who is already in her golden years, it is in your best interest to engage in some (or all) of these practices as much as possible. Good health, staying fit and strong, and enjoying longevity doesn't happen by accident. It requires conscious or deliberate actions.

Get involved in weight loss programs! While many diet programs may lead to weight loss, some of them can be too demanding and restrictive. Sustaining weight loss may not be feasible if the method for achieving it is too tasking. A better alternative to help keep your weight healthy is intermittent fasting, especially if you make a lifestyle change rather than a rapid weight loss attempt. As you grow older, you must allow your body enough time to digest and use up enough energy from your meals before shoving down another meal. One of the more apparent benefits of intermittent fasting is weight loss. If you can maintain a healthy weight as you age, your chances of developing insulin resistance (and all its attendant problems) grow slimmer.

Getting older is not an excuse for living a non-active lifestyle. To enjoy your advanced years, a regimented exercise program should be a central part of your lifestyle. The good thing about working out is that you are not limited to just a gym membership. You will learn some simple but effective exercises you can perform at home with small equipment. For a woman above 50, the key to getting impressive results with exercises is not how difficult or tedious the workout routine is or the length of the workout. The key to success with exercise is consistency even if it is a low-impact exercise, which I highly recommend. Performing exercises at least 30 minutes a day can greatly reduce your risk of developing insulin resistance.

Rest and quality sleep are also a big part of healthy living. It is not necessarily true that sleep declines as a person grows older. You still need between 7 and 8 hours of restful sleep even as you grow older. Without adequate sleep, your chances of developing high blood sugar levels increases. To give you an idea, scientists say that one sleepless night and an entire six months of a high-fat diet can mess with insulin sensitivity at almost the same rate (Science Daily, 2015).

Other Important Hormones That Can Impact Your Weight

Cortisol - The Stress Hormone

When your body senses stress, your adrenal glands release the hormone cortisol to help you deal with the stress. However, if you put your body through continued stress such as prolonged fasting or stringent diets over a long period, it can lead to a chronically elevated level of cortisol which is a situation you don't want to find yourself in. This situation can cause overeating and significant weight gain. One study showed that women who followed a low-calorie diet had increased cortisol levels and also felt more stressed than their counterparts on a normal diet (Tomiyama, et. al., 2010). To reduce cortisol levels, and by extension, adverse response to stress, engage in activities that soothe you, such as uninterrupted sleep, spending time with loved ones, and meditation. During your fasting window, it is a good practice to create time to meditate or at least listen to soothing music as this can decrease cortisol levels.

Leptin - The Satiety Hormone

Leptin is produced mainly in your fat cells. When you eat, leptin tells your brain when you have had enough. This instruction makes you think it's time to stop eating. But instead of high levels of leptin in the body to reduce your appetite, it works the other way round. The higher your leptin, the more you will eat. This is an indication of resistance and works similar to insulin resistance. Too much leptin means that your brain is not receiving the 'you are full' instruction. So your brain assumes you are still hungry even if you are overeating and have more than enough energy in storage.

Weight loss can help you maintain a normal leptin level. Getting adequate body movement through exercise, in addition to quality sleep, can help to boost your leptin sensitivity. By including fatty fish and more of other anti-inflammatory foods in your meals can help improve leptin sensitivity. Avoid excessive calorie restriction as this can deprive your body of vital nutrients and disrupt the production of hormones. Once your hormones are disrupted, it can lead to slower metabolism as well as mess with leptin levels.

Ghrelin - The Hunger Hormone

Ghrelin is triggered when your stomach is empty. It tells your brain that you need to eat, and makes you start feeling hungry. Usually, your ghrelin level is at its peak when you are hungry and drops significantly after your meal. But in obese people, ghrelin

16

levels only decrease slightly after meals. This means that their brains aren't flagged to stop and they often end up consuming too much.

A good way to deal with this hormone problem is to limit or avoid sugar-sweetened drinks as they can weaken your ghrelin response after a meal. Having adequate protein in your meals can also help. This is why it is best to eat clean when you fast intermittently. You're doing your health goals any favors by fasting for long hours only to eat junk when it really needs nutrients and vitamins.

Neuropeptide Y (NPY) - The Appetite Hormone

The Neuropeptide Y hormone is produced by brain cells and those in the nervous system. It stimulates appetite, especially those pesky cravings for carbohydrates that never seem to be satiated. The hormone is highest when you go without food, as done with fasting. Elevated levels of NPY can result in overeating and abdominal fat gain. An effective way to maintain healthy levels of NPY is to avoid fasting for too long. Engaging in prolonged fasting (over 24 hours) can significantly increase NPY levels.

Age-Related Issues

For many postmenopausal women – mostly women in their late 60s and early 70s – the issue is not so much about weight gain as it is about frailness, risk of chronic diseases, a lack of vigor, and a host of other factors that can cut short longevity and put their health on a downward spiral.

Medications may offer temporary relief, but are the unpleasant side effects worth it? Are women doomed to a life of discomfort, soreness, irritation, and an inevitable decline in vitality as they age? For many women who can't seem to see a satisfactory solution, the future appears dark and full of anxiety. This notion may be largely responsible for why some women dread growing old. They obsess unnecessarily with staying young and would put their bodies through unnecessarily complicated diets just to remain healthy and strong as they age. Unfortunately, a lot of women give up on stringent diets and other difficult lifestyle changes that promise vitality and longevity.

As a woman, you can age gracefully without medications or following some exacting lifestyle changes. All you need is modifying your eating pattern as introduced. But before you start making changes to the timing of your meals, it is important to heed the series of suggestions already given in this chapter to avoid possible negative impacts on your system. Even women of childbearing age can be negatively impacted by fasting because anything affecting a woman's reproductive hormones can certainly impact her overall health and wellbeing. And although most women over 50 are generally not looking to have kids, fasting can still disrupt body function.

Intermittent Fasting for Women Over 50

Intermittent fasting is not only safe but it is a very healthy practice for women over 50. Middle-aged and older women can gain a lot more than weight loss from fasting intermittently. In fact, the impact of intermittent fasting on cellular health is a key strategy for longevity, especially for older women.

When you stay away from food for longer periods than your body is used to, you allow your cells to carry out their natural function of detoxifying and cleaning themselves. During the series of metabolic activities that take place in your body, a lot of accumulated debris is left behind. Fasting helps to get rid of the debris and cause regeneration. A kind of reset.

As mentioned before, positive stressors are what you want. Intermittent fasting induces positive stress in a similar way exercises do to the body. By breaking down and rebuilding muscles, exercises make your muscles stronger and resilient. In the same way, staying away from food for longer than usual periods can put positive stressors on your body and help in the following ways:

1.   Resets circadian rhythms : The circadian rhythm is your internal clock that regulates almost every bodily process. Negative stress can disrupt the internal clock and lead to a host of negative effects, including sleep disorders. One common cause of circadian rhythm disruption is menopause. But menopausal and postmenopausal women who practice intermittent fasting can enjoy the benefit of a regular-functioning internal clock.

2.   Improves heart function : The heart cells can require high energy to function properly. Besides carbs, fat, and amino acids, the energy needs of your heart cells can be supplied through ketones activated by fasting. Ketones help to optimize your heart's

performance. It can also protect your heart from injury and inflammation.

3.   Reboots your gut flora : Intermittent fasting helps your gut health and your digestive system to reboot. This reset should happen regularly as the health of your digestive system determines the performance of your immune system. Also, your mood and mental health are connected to the health of your gut flora.

4.   Improves brain function : When you fast, ketones are produced to fuel your brain. Ketones generate fewer injurious reactive oxygen species (ROS). This means your brain performs better when it is powered by ketones instead of glucose.

Intermittent fasting, when practiced correctly, can act as maintenance of your body's various systems. Keep in mind that intermittent fasting is a pattern of eating, not stop and start eating. It is incomplete without proper re-feeding. Many of the "miracles" of fasting actually take place during the period of reintroducing food after cellular cleansing during the fasting period. So don't deprive yourself of healthy and normal-sized meals after fasting and remember to give up snacking, especially after dinner. To make your systems harmonize, you must synchronize. Nights are meant for sleeping, and your circadian system is cued for that. If you snack after dinner, it can throw your circadian system out of sync and mess with your natural ability to repair.

Listen to Your Body

As a woman over 50, you don't need to try very hard to know

what your body is telling you. The advice to pay attention to your body, is necessary for younger women in particular because some of them may not treat their body the best or know what their hormones are signaling. By the time a woman gets to 50, she is well aware of how her body communicates.

Nevertheless, it is possible to assume that what works for one healthy woman is also working for others in her age group and on the same health level. As much as it is important to engage in practices that keep you healthy, you need to pay attention to how you feel inside because that is how your hormones tell you what is working for you. Keep tabs on hormonal health because that is one of the greatest risks women of all ages face when they fast. It is not just estrogen and other sex hormones that are important. Your thyroid, cortisol, and follicle-stimulating hormones (FSH) all need to be at equilibrium or near-perfect balance as much as possible.

Your hormones may respond negatively to excessive stress that can be caused by combining intermittent fasting with dieting. It doesn't matter if you know someone who successfully combined fasting and dieting. What matters is what your body tells you. Staying fit and healthy should be fun and not feel like punishment. As a woman in her golden years, if you have decided to try intermittent fasting, I suggest that you focus only on intermittent fasting to the exclusion of dieting.

CHAPTER 3
HOW INTERMITTENT FASTING
WORK

Intermittent fasting is the technique of scheduling your dishes for your body to obtain the most out of them. Rather than minimizing your calorie use in fifty percent, refuting yourself of all the foods you value, or diving right into a classy diet plan pattern, Intermittent fasting is an all-natural, logical, as well as healthy and balanced and also balanced method of eating that advertises fat burning. There are tons of ways to approach Intermittent Fasting.

It's defined as an eating pattern. This technique focuses on altering when you take in, instead of what you consume.

When you begin Intermittent fasting, you will be more than likely to maintain your calorie intake the same; nonetheless, in contrast to spreading your dishes throughout the day, you will undoubtedly eat more significant recipes throughout a much shorter amount of time. As opposed to consuming 3 to 4 meals a day, you might eat one big meal at 11 am, afterward an added large dish at 6 pm, without any dine-in between 11 am as well as 6 pm, as well as also after 6 pm, no meal up until 11 am the adhering to day. This is simply one strategy of recurring fasting, and likewise, others will be-examined in this book in later stages.

Intermittent Fasting is a technique used by whole lots of bodybuilders, specialist athletes, and also physical health and fitness masters to maintain their muscular tissue mass high and their body fat percent reduced. Recurring fasting can be done short term or long term, but the very best results originate from embracing this technique right into your everyday lifestyle.

The word "fasting" might stress the average person; Intermittent fasting does not associate with starving yourself. To comprehend the principals behind effective Intermittent fasting, we'll at first review the body's digestion state: the fed state as well as the fasting state.

For 3 to 5 hours after consuming a meal, your body remains in what is described as the "fed state." Throughout the fed state, your insulin levels rise to soak up and digest your meal. When your insulin levels get high, it is exceptionally tough for your body to shed fat. Insulin is a hormone produced by the pancreatic to handle sugar degrees in the bloodstream. Its purpose is to manage insulin is technically a hormonal storage agent. When insulin degrees come to be so high, your body starts shedding your food for energy instead of your conserved fat. Which is why boosted degrees of it protect against weight reduction.

After the 3 to 5 hrs are up, your body has, in fact, finished refining the dish, and also you enter the post-absorptive state. The post-absorptive state lasts anywhere from 8 to 12 hours. When your body comes, hereafter the time room is the fasted state. As a result of the reality that your body has refined your food by this.

Factor, your insulin levels are reduced, making you kept fat extremely available for losing.

Persisting fasting allows your body to get to an innovative weight loss state that you would usually obtain to with the average' 3 meals daily' eating pattern. They are just altering the timing as well as the pattern of their food intake. It may take some time to get when you start an Intermittent Fasting program right into the swing of points. Merely obtain back if you slip up right into your Intermittent fasting pattern when you can.

Making a way of living adjustment entails a purposeful initiative, and also no one expects you to do it completely today. Intermittent fasting will definitely take some getting used to if you are not in the practice of going long periods without eating. As long as you pick the right technique for you, continue to be focused, and also remain concentrated, you will unanimously grasp it quickly.

Unlike some of the other diet regimen strategy that you may embark on, the Intermittent fast is one that will certainly work. When you listen to, it is simple to obtain a bit terrified regarding fasting.

Recurring fasting is a little bit various than you might assume. If you finish up being on, your body will often go right into hunger mode, the rapid for as well lengthy.

You do not need to get as well concerned about exactly how this Intermittent quickly will work in the cravings mode. The Intermittent fast is efficient because you are not going to quick for as long that the body gets in right into this malnourishment setting as well as stops minimizing weight. Instead, it will make the rapid continue long enough that you will have the ability to accelerate the metabolic process.

With the Intermittent quick, you will discover that when you opt for a couple of hrs without eating (usually no more than 2 - 4 hrs), the body is not going to go right into malnourishment setting. When complying with a recurring fasting plan, you require your body to melt more fat without placing in any sort-of extra job.

Here are a couple of fast pointers for success:

Mostly, it is essential not to expect to see outcomes from your new lifestyle promptly. Perhaps, you need to focus on devoting to the process for a minimum of 30 days before you can start to evaluate the results correctly.

Second, it is imperative to remember that the excellent quality of the food you place into your body still matters as it will certainly merely take a few convenience food meals to reverse all of your tough work.

For the excellent results, you will plan to consist of an in-light exercise routine during quick days along with a far more fundamental regimen for full-calorie days.

Recurring Fasting describes nutritional consuming patterns that include not consuming or continuos limiting calories for a long term period, Intermittent Fasting (. There are various subgroups of regular fastings each with variance in the duration of the fast of individuals, some for hrs, others for day(s). This has finished up being an extremely liked subject in the clinical research area as a result of every one of the prospective advantages of fitness in addition to health that is being found.

The diet regimen you adhere to whilst Recurring Fasting will be figured out by the results that you are looking for as well as where you are beginning with additionally, so take a look at on your own and ask the question what do I want from this?

If you are looking for to lose a significant quantity of weight, then you are mosting likely to have to take a look at your diet regimen plan extra closely, yet if you wish to shed a couple of pounds for the beach, then you could discover that a pair of weeks of Recurring fasting can do that for you.

There are many various ways you can do recurring fasting. We just are most likely to consider the 24-hour fasting system in which is what I used to shed 27 pounds over a 2-month duration. You could really feel some cravings pains, but these will pass also, as you end up being even more familiar with Intermittent fasting you might find as I have that feeling of need no more existing you with a concern.

While fasting, it is suggested to drink a lot of water to avoid coffee, tea and dehydration are fine as long as you take a sprinkle of milk. If you are fretted that you are not getting adequate nutrients into your body, then you might consider a juice made from celery, lime, broccoli, and also ginger, which will taste fantastic and also get some sufficient nutrient fluid into your body. It would be best to stick to the coffee, water, and tea if you can handle it.

Whatever your diet strategy is whether it's healthy or not you should see weight reduction after regarding three weeks of Intermittent Fasting as well as do not be put off if you do not find much advancement at first, it's not a race, and also it is much far better to drop weight in a straight style over time as opposed to collision losing a couple of extra pounds which you will put right back on. After the initial month, you might want to have an appearance at your diet plan on non-fasting days and also remove high sugar foods and even any scrap that you might generally take in. I have discovered that intermittent fasting over the long-term tends to make me wish to consume healthier foods as an all-natural routine.

If you are practicing intermittent fasting for bodybuilding, then you may wish to consider having a look at your macro-nutrients and also working out just how much healthy protein as well as carbohydrate you call for to eat, this is a lot more complex, as well as you can uncover info about this on several websites which you will need to spend time examining for the very best end results.

There are great deals of advantages to recurring fasting, which you will view as you proceed, a few of these advantages include even more energy, much less bloating, a clearer mind, and a basic feeling of wellness. It's important not to succumb to any type of lure to binge eat after a fasting duration, as this will negate the influence obtained from the recurring fasting period.

In verdict simply by adhering to a two times a week 24-hour Intermittent Fasting approach for a couple of weeks you will slim down however if you can boost your diet plan on the days that you do not rapid then you will lose more weight and if you can remain with this system, then you will certainly keep the weight off without turning to any kind of fad diet regimen or diet plans that are difficult to stick to.

CHAPTER 4
WHY INTERMITTENT FASTING IS IDEAL FOR WOMEN OVER 50

Improved Mental Concentration and Clarity

Fasting has incredible benefits for the healthy function of the brain. The most known benefit stems from the activation of autophagy, which is a cell cleansing process. Note that fasting has anti-seizure effects.

Improvement in Hormone Profile

There are plenty of people who avoid intermittent fasting as they feel it will cause their fitness levels to deteriorate. This isn't necessarily the case for those people who do take part in intermittent fasting, as studies have shown that fasting does not negatively impact those who perform regular physical activities, especially if you cut down on your carbs as you fast and are in a ketosis state. Studies have shown that physical training while fasting can lead to higher metabolic adaptations.

Reduces Inflammation

Intermittent fasting promotes autophagy, a process in which the body destroys its old or damaged cells. Killing off old cells may sound like a terrible notion. However, it can be seen as a way of removing old and unwanted dirt from your body. It's a simple method for the body to clean and repair itself. Old and damaged cells can create inflammation. Because intermittent fasting stimulates autophagy, then it is possible to reduce inflammation in your body while fasting.

Supports Healthy Bodily Functions

Intermittent fasting gives your body time to complete processes and functions before introducing more food into your system. This means that every time you eat, you are giving your body adequate time to actually metabolize the food and use it appropriately. In modern society, we regularly overeat and push our bodies to constantly be in a state of digesting. As a result, our systems become overwhelmed and we do not effectively metabolize everything. This can lead to you not getting enough nutrition, storing fats, and struggling to produce healthy levels of natural hormones and chemicals within your body.

Polycystic Ovarian Syndrome and Intermittent Fasting

Polycystic ovaries are a fairly common disease in women. This disease causes a hormone shift and can have any undesirable effects on women. Many women struggle with weight gain and difficulty losing weight as a side effect of the disease. While there are not very many studies about how intermittent fasting affects the disease, there is evidence that combining intermittent fasting with a keto diet significantly helped to regulate the hormones and made weight loss possible for polycystic ovarian syndrome patients. There does seem to be some potential hope with using intermittent fasting to help treat and maintain diseases like polycystic ovarian syndrome and other hormonal disorders. Time and additional research will tell us if intermittent fasting has a future in helping with this disease.

Metabolic Reset

Many women, as they age, experience reduced metabolism. This is partly due to the natural aging process, and partly due to damaging the metabolism over the decades. Frequent crash dieting, poor sleep, overworking, poor health, and more can all damage your metabolism, thus preventing you from losing weight. But, by merely practicing intermittent fasting, you can reset and boost your metabolism, not only allowing you to lose weight but also helping you to feel healthier and maintain healthy lean muscle as you age.

Change in Cell Function

When you fast for a while, different changes take place in your body. For instance, your body will start a process of cellular repair and there will be changes in your hormone level. A difference in these levels makes it easier for the body to access the stored fat. You will notice that there is a reduction in the level of insulin and it helps increase the body's ability to burn fat. An increase in the human growth hormone helps to increase lean muscle and burn more fat than usual. Damaged cells are processed and other processes of cellular repair kick in. In addition, several changes take place within the genes and molecules that protect you against disease.

Improved Sleep

In the paragraph above, it was mentioned that sometimes efforts to lose weight are undermined by insufficient sleep. There has been at least one scientific study which has shown that people who persist with intermittent fasting for a year or more have better sleep. The reasons why this occurs are no doubt complicated, but there have been conclusive demonstrations that intermittent fasting over an extended period assists good sleep.

Mood and Motivation

The study of the effect of intermittent fasting on mood and motivation is in its infancy. There is a lack of research on large populations, using the statistical techniques of randomized controls. However, some studies have demonstrated that intermittent fasting does improve both mood and motivation in a surprisingly short period. As there is profound controversy about the pharmacological treatments of people's mental state, any treatment which has no side effects and many potential benefits must be considered seriously.

Cardiovascular Health

Intermittent fasting leads to a reduction in weight. For this and other reasons, it leads to an improvement in cardiovascular health. The cause of such disease is usually atherosclerosis, the deposit of plaque in blood vessel walls. The dysfunction of the endothelium, which is a thin lining of the blood vessels, causes atherosclerosis. A healthy endothelium works to prevent this insidious deposit. The endothelium is not doing its job properly if plaque builds up.

Obesity, especially where the fat deposits are in the abdominal area, leads in many cases to this buildup of plaque.

Other causes of this deposit are stress and inflammation. Intermittent fasting assists in the reduction of these, as well as obesity. Some studies show improvements in all risk factors for cardiovascular health.

Gut Health

Increasingly, scientists are becoming ever more aware that microorganisms living in the human gut or digestive system perform vital functions. These are known as the microbiome. There are trillions of them and they are in other parts of the body, apart from the gut. Many diseases originate in the gut, not only illnesses concerning that part of the body, but also of the brain, the heart, and all other regions of the body.

There is research on mice that caloric restriction improves that part of the microbiome in the gut. The effect of this is to prolong the life of the mice. In humans, the effects of dietary changes are very swift, even as short as hours. Studies are currently being done to verify that the real effects of intermittent fasting observed in the gut health of mice are true for humans as well.

Weight Loss

The most obvious benefit of this diet is weight loss. When you follow intermittent fasting, the number of meals you eat will be reduced. When you eat less, the calories you consume will decrease as well. When the levels of insulin decline, growth hormone increases along with an increase in norepinephrine, which helps the body break down stored fat to provide energy. There is an increase in your metabolic rate when you fast, which helps the body burn more calories. The effect of intermittent fasting is two-fold. On the one hand, it increases your metabolic rate and therefore makes your body more efficient while burning fats. The reduction in the level of food you consume reduces your overall calorie intake.

Lower the Risk of Diabetes

The most common health problem that plagues humanity these days, apart from obesity, is diabetes. High blood sugar leads to insulin resistance in the body. Intermittent fasting helps to reduce blood sugar and therefore helps reduce insulin resistance in the body. When your body becomes resistant to insulin, it leads to an increase in the blood sugar level and the vicious cycle goes on and on. If you opt for this diet, you can successfully reverse this condition.

It boosts your metabolic rate

Studies show that staying in a fasted state leads to a spike in the hormone norepinephrine. This hormone increases your basal metabolic rate and burns fat. On top of that, once you enter your eating window, your metabolism still stays at an elevated level. You are essentially burning excess fat even when eating!

Convert Your Body Fat

Many people are unaware, but there are two types of body fat, white and brown. This fat is not created equal. Just as there is healthy and unhealthy cholesterol, there is also sturdy and unhealthy body fat. The white fat, which is what builds up as people gain excess weight, is damaging to health, contributes to aging, and leads to disease.

On the other hand, brown body fat is vital in protecting the body's inner organs and maintaining health. When you practice intermittent fasting, it not only helps you lose weight, but it can also actively convert your unhealthy white fat to healthy brown fat. As if that weren't good enough, brown fat also helps burn off white fat, meaning that the more brown fat you have, the more you will burn off excess white body fat.

Improve Muscle Health

Many people get excited about the temporary weight reduction they experience when trying the crash diet. That is until they stop losing weight and eventually give up on a diet. But, most of the weight loss people achieve on these diets is not fat loss but water weight and muscle weight. Muscle weighs more than fat, so even a small amount of muscle loss can make a big difference on the scale.

As crash diets promote malnutrition, it naturally leads to muscle loss, which negatively affects your health and strength as you age. After all, your muscles are in much more than your arms. They are surrounding your entire body, and even your heart is a muscle! As you lose muscle, your health and energy will be dramatically affected, and it is essential to regain this as you age if you want to improve your health. Thankfully, studies have found that when compared to dieting, intermittent fasting not only leads to more weight loss than dieting, but it also causes much less muscle loss. This means your muscles will become much healthier, especially if you actively workout while you practice fasting.

Boosted Energy

The mitochondria, which are within our mitochondrial cells, are the powerhouse of the cell. It is the mitochondria that allow us to use a variety of fuel sources from the food we eat as fuel, as well as ketones. While other cells in the body may only be able to utilize one or two fuel types for energy, the mitochondrial is incredibly versatile to be able to use all kinds of fuel. When you fast for longer periods (or are on a low-carb/ketogenic diet), your body begins to produce ketones, which are then used to cross the blood-brain barrier and fuel the brain in the absence of glucose. But that is not all. When you are in this fasted state of ketosis, the body will also increase the number of mitochondrial cells within your body, replacing non-mitochondrial cells with mitochondrial cells, allowing for more of your cells to be fueled by any fuel source.

Since the mitochondrial fuel ninety percent of the human body, by increasing the number of these cells, you can naturally increase your energy. Not only will your physical energy increase, but your mental functioning and energy will, as well. This is great news for many people who lose energy as they age.

Reduce Insulin Resistance

Insulin is perhaps the most well-known hormone, as the number of people diagnosed with diabetes only continues to rise. But insulin does not only affect people with diabetes but for everyone. This hormone, produced by the pancreas, is released after eating to allow the cells to absorb and utilize glucose as an energy source. But, often, our sensitivity to insulin decreases as we age or put on weight. The cells can become resistant to insulin, which leads to them being unable to absorb the glucose we have ingested. Over time, this causes a buildup of glucose in the bloodstream and, ultimately, diabetes if it is left untreated.

However, whether you have insulin resistance or already have been diagnosed with type II diabetes, you don't have to allow your condition to worsen. You can treat your insulin resistance directly at the source, and in the process, improve the absorption of glucose by your cells. Many people can lower the severity of their insulin resistance or diabetes, and some are even able to treat it completely.

Multiple controlled studies have found that intermittent fasting can both treat insulin resistance and lower blood glucose levels. Some studies have found that intermittent fasting can even be as effective, if not more effective, than dieting for lowering blood glucose levels.

Increase Neural Cells

It is important to take care of brain health as we age, especially as the levels of Alzheimer's disease, Parkinson's disease, and other neurodegenerative diseases are on the rise. But, one way that intermittent fasting can help guard against and treat all brain-related diseases is by increasing the production and repair of neural cells. This is important, as these diseases all cause these vital brain cells to become damaged or stunted overtime.

The result is that if you begin practicing intermittent fasting regularly now, you can reduce your risk of developing a neurological disease in the future. Or, if you already have one, you may be able to reduce symptoms or halt its progression. This is amazing news, as neurological diseases are incredibly hard to treat, even with modern medicine. Studies have specifically shown intermittent fasting to increase cell growth and repair in the cortex, hippocampus, basal forebrain, and nervous system. Along with the decreased risk of disease and disease progression, you can also expect to experience increased mental energy, better focus, improved memory, and a stabilized mood.

Lessen Oxidative Stress

Toxins cause oxidative stress. We can develop these toxins when we breathe in poor quality air, don't sleep well, eat poor quality food, apply damaging substances to our skin, and much more. We even develop this oxidative stress when our cells convert fuel to energy, meaning that even if we live in a clean environment, sleep perfectly, and only eat organic food, we would still develop oxidative stress, thereby causing damage to our cells. As our cells develop this damage from oxidative stress, we slowly lose our health and energy, producing an increased risk of disease.

However, studies have shown that intermittent fasting not only increases the rate our cells develop oxidative stress, but it also increases our body's natural antioxidants to fight against this damage directly.

Improve Mental Well-Being

Poor mental health is becoming more common than ever, with over forty-million Americans suffering from one form of mental illness or another, and many others struggling with short-term depression and anxiety. One of the most common causes of disability in middle-aged Americans (as well as those who are young) is chronic severe depression. Yet, a majority of these people never seek professional help.

While I urge you always to seek professional help for your mental health, you can also practice intermittent fasting. Studies have found that with short-term fasting, people can significantly improve their everyday mood, tranquility, alertness, and even the feeling of euphoria. Not only that but also the symptoms of severe depression can be improved with fasting.

Treat or Prevent Disease

While we cannot guarantee that intermittent fasting will prevent you from developing a disease or treat an infection you already have, many studies have proven that fasting can help. These studies have shown that fasting a person can menage their symptoms, possibly reverse the condition, and significantly reduce your likelihood of ever developing a disease. Now that we have looked at the general ways in which intermittent fasting can improve your health, let's have a look at some of the specific diseases and conditions you can expect short-term fasting to improve.

Less food consumption

One of the things you will notice over time is that you will begin to consume less food within your feasting window. Try to examine your food portions during your intermittent fast, and you'll see this clearly. Research shows that when fasting, you end up consuming 20% less food than the period before you began fasting. This is possibly due to the levels of the ghrelin hormone being normalized. Ghrelin is responsible for controlling appetite and triggering hunger, and in most of us, this hormone doesn't function efficiently. Due to our modern diet, a lot of our hormones are out of sync, which is why we feel hungry and eat all the time. Once your ghrelin starts working properly, you will feel less hungry.

It slows down the progression of cancer.

A study conducted on mice at the Duke University Medical Center in North Carolina showed that the caloric deficit resulting from intermittent fasting actually slowed down cancer in the mice.

Reduces Inflammation

Oxidative stress is one of the main reasons for inflammation in the body. Inflammation is the body's natural reaction to illness. However, excess inflammation is a painful condition and causes a host of diseases like arthritis. When the unstable molecules in the body, known as free radicals, react with other essential molecules like proteins and DNA, it causes inflammation. Intermittent fasting helps reduce inflammation and also offers protection against aging. Premature aging isn't desirable, now is it?

Heart's Health

Heart disease is the most significant killer in the world. Several risk factors increase the chance of heart disease. Intermittent fasting helps reduce risk factors like blood pressure, high cholesterol, inflammatory markers, blood sugar and blood triglycerides. When you can control these risk factors, you reduce the chance of suffering from cardiovascular disease. However, once again, a lot of research in this field is based on animal studies.

Cellular Repair

Autophagy is the process of waste removal in the body, and intermittent fasting helps to kick-start this process. The body breaks down and metabolizes broken, as well as dysfunctional, proteins. An increase in autophagy protects you from several degenerative diseases like cancer and Alzheimer's.

All these benefits help to increase your lifespan and help you lead a healthier life. Not only will you lose weight, but you can also improve your overall health just by following the intermittent fasting method.

Supports You in Healing Faster

When your cells have an easier time restoring themselves and your body is exposed to less stress, you have an easier time in healing faster. This means that any time you place a physical strain on your body, you can look forward to spending less time healing from that experience.

May Extend Your Lifespan

Intermittent fasting has shown in some studies that it may be able to extend your lifespan. Many people find themselves living shorter lives with poorer quality of life as a result of poor health. Disease and illness kill far more people each year than actual old age or natural causes do. Using the intermittent fasting diet may support you in preventing these illnesses and diseases so that you can live a longer, healthier, natural life.

Boosts Your Immune System

As a result of the many benefits that you gain from intermittent fasting, you also get to look forward to having an improved immune system. This is from the combination of reduced physical stress, increased cellular reparation abilities, weight loss, and other benefits that you gain from intermittent fasting.

Improved Sex Drive

Lower levels of production in both estrogen and testosterone may lead to a decreased sex drive. As such, it is not a psychological or physiological issue, but it is a hormonal matter. So, when you engage in intermittent fasting, your brain will regain its balance and begin to produce the right levels of all hormones.

So, in addition to improving your cognitive ability, restricting the production of cortisol, and boosting your mood through increased production of endorphins and dopamine, your body will also regulate the production of estrogen and testosterone which could potentially lead to a healthier sex drive.

Cellular Repair

Autophagy is the process of waste removal in the body, and intermittent fasting helps to kick-start this process. The body breaks down and metabolizes broken, as well as dysfunctional, proteins. An increase in autophagy protects you from several degenerative diseases like cancer and Alzheimer's.

All these benefits help to increase your lifespan and help you lead a healthier life. Not only will you lose weight, but you can also improve your overall health just by following the intermittent fasting method.

CHAPTER 5
INTERMITTENT FASTING TYPES FOR WOMEN OVER 50

When discussing the types of intermittent fasting, it is vital to remember that there is no one size fits all. There is really no need to look for that one perfect method that will suit you. Even among the methods that exist, the intermittent fasting an always be modified and adapted to your lifestyle. It exists as an adaptation of your naturally healthy lifestyle, not the other way around.

The main difference between different methods is clearly the time window in which you can eat and skip the meals. Some fast for a longer time because their body can easily take it. As a woman in fifties, you will either find fasting improving your skin, giving you better digestion along with metabolism and such, or it will not suit you at all. Listen to your body. Does it experience stress after fasting? Does it experience mild pressure on your shoulders or irregular periods? The intermittent fasting is really not for you if it does.

The best thing about the methods of intermittent fasting is that they are flexible. Not only can you adapt them to your life style, you can also change them into your own way. Like I have said before that skipping breakfast and eating at noon is not the strictly right way. Everybody does their own way and that is quite amazing. Does your body naturally remain healthy with daylight eating cycle? Don't skip your breakfast then! No good comes from that! Similarly, when you read these methods, you will want to make sure that some of the information is given as a general one. Most of the restrictions are on time and well, time can always be adjusted. Try the different methods and see for yourself which one is the right way. Like I have said, listen to your body.

The intermittent fasting would require you to seek the advice of medical health professional if you had a stomach issues or you are pregnant.

1.   16/8 Method:

16/8 method has been talked about before frequently. You are quite familiar with it by now. The 16/8 method allows you to set a time window of eight hours for food consumption. Later, you will be fasting for the rest of 16 hours.

The simplest and trendiest way to do it is skipping the breakfast and eating the meal at 1 pm or noon. Then, as the time would pass, you would need to consume your next meal within next eight hours. Preferably, you should eat at first hour of eight hours window. Then, you should eat at the last hour of eight hours window. So, you would have to move forward with this.

Most people eat their first meal around 1 pm, then 5 pm and then fast for the rest of the day. With proper nutrition and calories, this is quite possible. Some people go around with eating at noon and then eating their next meal at dinner time. This would also work brilliantly provided you are meeting the right calorie demands. Furthermore, it is worth noting that this procedure doesn't require you to skip your breakfast.

There is a negative talk about the 16/8 method since people have specified it with idea of skipping breakfast. Mostly online articles will tell you how intermittent fasting means skipping the breakfast and then moving on with the day.

As a fifty years old woman or someone near that age, if you have spent your life never skipping breakfast then it isn't wise to do it now. You can easily make room for your intermittent fasting by having your breakfast, then your lunch and then skipping the meal for the rest of the day. Please know that even this can be adjusted. You don't need to start having breakfast early if you are a late morning eater. Really all you need to do is to adjust your time window of eight hour of eating and sixteen hours of fasting.

Interestingly, for beginners and busy adults, this is a preferred method. If you are a working lady, this method would easily suit you. For a working lady in her fifties or forties, the intermittent fasting is very much the preferred method of diet. Why? Some of the busy women already skip their breakfast due to a tight schedule. I have seen plenty of such cases. Therefore, by intermittent fasting they are simply adjusting their schedule to one that of healthy lifestyle.

Similarly, for some women, the intermittent fasting is right method as beginners. Why? Because it suits them quite a lot. Some women may not feel hungry at dinner time because they already might have heavy meals near breakfast and lunch. In such case, intermittent fasting is already a confirmed choice.

The 16/8 fasting method may not work for everyone. Why? Some women's natural body cycles are not accustomed to it. They can still do it but not by sticking strictly to the eight hours restriction. You can extend it to flexible hours range. This type of intermittent fasting is perfect for losing weight. In truth, when you go on this type of fast, there is one special benefit. The science has shown when you limit the eating window to eight hours, you automatically consume lesser calories. Even if you are eating the same amount of calories on everyday basis, the amount of calories consumption is automatically increased to a good limit. This will end up burning more calories on same calorie intake than before. Thus, if you can stick with this plan, it would actually be best. It suits especially those people who want to try a dieting pattern while not being able to go a specific diet or their routine is too busy. Interestingly, this kind of fasting is also more assistive in providing resistance against the disease. It certainly helps against the obesity and diabetes as well as inflammation. As a fifty years old woman or someone near, if you manage to make it work then it will benefit you the most. Take care that when your body changes or is undergoing through several cycles, you will need to consult your health professional. All in all, it is a great technique.

2. 12 Hours Fasting

This is the kind of fasting some of us automatically do and reap its benefits. For females who are starting as new, it would benefit them to start with this method. Most of your time is spent in sleeping so you will not have to worry about hunger pangs. In fact, many people start with this kind of fasting and slowly switch to the advanced forms later. Some people find the perfect balance of exercise and this type of fasting.

The best thing about this particular type of intermittent fasting is that it doesn't restrict your exercise schedule. You can pair up heavy cardio with this type of intermittent fasting and actually get good results.

The mechanism behind this approach is same as the ones like it. The thing about this wonderful method is that it doesn't need to be switched. It has the most chance of working out for women because it doesn't require you start making serious sacrifices on your schedule. You can first eat at 7 am or 8 am. You should then eat the next meal before 8 pm and then let the day pass. You can find it easy to integrate this into your daily life. It doesn't make sudden drastic changes in your life that you will find uncomfortable to keep. Interestingly, the body calories are consumed more than they are stored as fats. Therefore, the calories are consumed more often as compared to regular eating method. This will lead to weight loss. As I have explained before, since most time is spent in sleeping, it is automatically a favorite for people. Some women find this system so amazing that they don't move beyond the 12 hours fast technique. They have perfectly managed to make it work and chances are you will too!

As I have already explained, this is a method that is least painful to follow. If you find that intermittent fasting gives you acidity or that sixteen hours fast is not cutting it for you, feel free to switch to this method. I am sure it will be much easier.

There are several added benefits of 12 hour fasting. Note that these benefits are most visible when you start out as new. These benefits will increase once you increase that time of fasting. However, the most visible benefits are when you switch from no fasting to that of 12 hours fasting.

The first change that you will observe would be of brain efficiency. Your brain functions will be enhanced than usual. The next thing that you are going to notice while following a 12 hours fast is that of detoxification. This is something that you will want to be on a look out for. You will need to see what is genuine detoxification and what is the side effect of the fasting. Some women mistake the signs of detoxification as possible side effects when your body is actually healing itself by removing waste. The last benefit is most obvious. It is that of weight loss since calorie intake is automatically reduced regardless of same calorie intake everyday.

3.   2 Days a Week/5:2 Diet

This is the most popular method of fasting. Many diet trends are set around this and a lot of people have achieved this with successful results. This method is also known as 5:2 method. Made famous by British journalist Michel Mosley, this method has set new trends. Like all other intermittent fasting approaches, there are many flexible variants of this.

Why is it called 5:2? If you look at the title of this section, it says 2 days a week. This is exactly what it sounds like. Out of seven days of week, two will be dedicated to the fasting. Some people restrict themselves to observe full-fledged fast on those two days. They take in minimum amount of calories like 500-600 calories a day. However, there is really no restriction on what to eat. However, the restriction is on when you will be eating your meal. This means there is no set amount of calories than should be taken on two days of fasting. If you are one of those women who find it easier to observe full-fledged fasts on two days of week without undergoing strict diet patterns, this is the technique for you.

The dieting pattern in this intermittent fasting approach is quite easily to be explained. For five days a week, you eat regularly like on normal days. For two days, you are going to observe fast. This automatically means that you will need to restrict the calorie intake. For women, usually it will be 500 calories for that day.

There should always be something that you should take care of. You should always have at least one non-fasting day between the fasting days. Select any two days you want to. Some people pick weekends. I personally like the idea. However, as long as your weekends are not going to be affected properly and there is a break of one non fasting day between, you are good to go.

There is also another thing that you need to take care of. Just because intermittent fasting doesn't place any restriction on eating, this doesn't mean you should start eating anything you would like to eat. If you do, you may end up sabotaging your fasting progress. Furthermore, please try not to eat too much at once. The purpose of fasting would be lost then. I have seen some people gaining weight which was opposite of what they wanted to achieve.

The health benefits of this approach are immense and impressive. If you find that this technique works for you, you will reap immense benefits. Weight loss is one of the benefits. The insulin resistance that helps fight off diabetes is also another benefit of this technique. The blood sugar levels are also regulated in some cases for people who have problems with them. Generally, all the fasting benefits can be reaped using this one approach in a short time.

4.   Alternate Day Fasting:

This is quite an advanced technique of intermittent fasting. In this technique, you fast one day and you pass your next day with normal eating. That is why it is called alternate day fasting. This is because you fast every other day and eat regular diet on other day. I suggest this method for advanced fasters who have quite practice with that. The alternate day fasting would not be recommended for the beginners. Even for adept women who have been fasting for some time, they can continue the alternate day fasting for some time.

Alternate day fasting can be a very powerful tool for weight loss. Unlike other approaches of fasting, this method can yield results quickly. It also helps fight off type-2 diabetes and it has proved to be quite effective against the heart diseases.

The basic idea is you fast one day and eat what you want the next day. You will be making huge changes and for a beginner, those changes will be uncomfortable. As a woman above fifty or near that age, you will need to consider the professional medical advice. If you have had good experience with fasting, then you can easily go for the alternate day fasting method.

You will only need to restrict what you eat half of the time. For example, one day might be the day of full scale meals (usually three). The next day can be the fasting day when you would consume as less calories as possible. You can try beverages on the fasting day as long as they are without calories. Water is one such beverage. The black tea and coffee that is unsweetened can be consumed as well. All in all, you should avoid taking in too many calories at once. Make sure on fasting, you eat only 25% of what you would eat on regular day.

Despite its advanced nature, it is quite an interesting fact that alternate day fasting is usually easier for people who are in the game. Those who find it difficult to have restriction on calories on everyday basis will find that alternate day is relatively easier. It might seem contradictory but if you cannot control your calorie intake during any meal, you can always skip the meal as part of fasting. The calorie intake is of course going to be reduced by this approach. You don't have to worry about gulping down specific portions when fasting will be reducing your calories automatically. Consuming limited calories on fasting day is far better than consuming nothing and doing a full fast.

You can also pair up the technique of alternate day fasting with endurance exercise. This will end up producing nearly twice the rate of fat loss, more muscle mass and cell growth. There is another wonderful aspect of alternate day fasting. Sometimes, we cannot choose between low fat diet and high fat diet. Alternate day fasting doesn't really care whether it is high fat or low fat meal you are consuming. Scientific studies showed that the alternate day fasting had similar results with both of the approaches. You can either eat the high fat diet or low fat diet and try out the alternate day fasting, both would have same results.

The alternate day fasting has an interesting effect on hunger. In some cases, the fasting approach is said to have decreased the hunger and made the body more tolerable to it. In some cases, the hunger remains same. In some cases however, the alternate day fasting will allow the hunger to be increased. This happens when you break the fast with oily foods and such. In my personal experience, I found that eating oily foods meant taking in more calories while increasing the hunger. Our body would start naturally craving those more and more. However, when the fast is broken with normal healthy diet such as rice or wheat bread, the body automatically fills up on lesser calories. This is the added advantage.

The most peculiar effect of intermittent fasting is that the muscle mass loses. The means your body starts toning itself more. The structure of natural healthy body is preserved and henceforth, this automatically means more weight loss. The muscle mass decrease means more fat loss and weight loss that will naturally lead to a slimmer body.

Interestingly, when body's natural state is preserved, the resistance against diseases is improved too in this fasting method. This means naturally those hormones are facilitated which are related to healthy functions of the body. The most prominent resistance that is developed is that of against the type 2 diabetes. The other resistance that is developed is against the heart diseases.

However, this must be kept in mind that if your body is compatible with fasting, then the alternate day fasting is for you. Make sure to consult the health professional.

5. Warrior Diet:

We are moving towards more advanced techniques of intermittent fasting as we are proceeding forward. The warrior diet is one of them. Before we start, the warrior diet has a negative impact on athletes and pregnant women. Therefore, I would strongly advise against warrior diet if you are any one of these. As a woman above fifty, I don't think you would be either so let me explain it in as simple terms as possible.

The warrior diet is something of a natural diet. It encourages our body to lose weight by its natural processes. Interestingly, to know the warrior diet, we would have to go back. The warrior diet is inspired from the ancient times. There were times when our human ancestors didn't lead a life as luxurious as we did. They had tight schedules to deal with and they didn't know things like we do.

Some of our ancestors didn't have time for a proper breakfast, a lunch and a well-settled dinner. They didn't have health professionals who told them of ways to lose weight. For our ancestors, the weight loss was not even a concern. Our ancestors or people of the old times followed one thing. They followed their instincts that guided them naturally.

Due to the busy schedule and day, they ate little to nothing during the day. However, at night, they feasted. It is basically a 20 hour fast in which you are eating nothing during the entire day but feasting at night. Night time is not considered the healthy time for a meal. I am a strong candidate of eating how much in this case scenario. If you have eaten nothing all day, then your body is starving. If you eat at night and you eat more than your regular meals, the body will not start gaining more weight. Unless you are only eating processed or oily foods, you shouldn't even be gaining fat. The fat is not going to appear from a magical place. Think about it! What you lacked during the entire day, you are eating at night. The calories are going to be balanced at night. The advice of not eating at night actually comes from the fact that your body cycle is least active at that time. For some people, the night time is the rest time. That is when their body is naturally less active. However, the natural body cycle of everyone differs. Secondly, if you have consumed calories all day, the body has already got enough supply of them. However, if you have not consumed them at all, the night time is not when those calories are going to be added as surplus. The surplus means more than enough. What you are feeding your body at night after entire day of fasting doesn't fall into category of surplus at all.

You have twenty hours window for fasting and four hours window for eating. In that four hourss window, naturally you will feast. For health concerns, I would recommend eating at least two to three hours before sleeping.

If you are a woman above fifty and your body adjusts to this fasting technique, you are going to appear as someone in her thirties or even lesser. I am not exaggerating. You will be very active trust me!

This method of fasting is quite advanced and it is not recommend for beginners at all. Unless you already have a good fasting experience, I wouldn't recommend taking a start from here. Furthermore, try it one day and see the results. If you are good to go, by all means proceed and make changes to your body.

There is one thing that should always be taken care of. Please remember to drink a lot of water. Your body is going to be dehydrated and this is going to be a tough experience. You will need to take in as much water as possible. Furthermore, to pass the day with ease, you can consume raw vegetables, fruits, eggs and dairy milk. You can also drink black tea or coffee. This is all going to be helpful while you pass the day while fasting. This can be a great way to increase the vegetable diet in your daily meals.

After the entire day has passed, you can actually eat as much as you want at night, provided it is not abnormally too much. The breaking of fast is also related to feasting which is taken as a literal term here. You are going to eat more than you eat on a regular meal. However, please eat regular foods. If you prepare oily foods and only eat delicious but high fat products, then this won't be much of a fast.

The warrior diet is really not a trend or a simple pattern. It is a lifestyle change that you will be making. Once you adapt, you will be easily making it a part of your life. If you change your body and switch to the warrior diet, you will end up losing weight fast. You can lose weight as much as hundred pounds or even more.

As long as you don't binge on unhealthy foods during the four hours window of eating, the warrior diet is going to be miraculous. I have found that when you consume the unhealthy foods, your body will crave more. The warrior diet is going to be difficult for you then. However, if you eat proper healthy foods during the warrior diet, you will find it easy to fast. Your body is going to consume the calories at a natural and healthy rate. Make sure you are following the healthy moderation. If you do that, there is nothing between you and the beneficial health effects.

One of the best changes that will be in your body is that you will not feel hunger at regular periods. The body will feel naturally balanced, requiring less.

The body is supposed to be changed slowly. You must give your body time. If you had success with fasting, please give your body time to recover. I say this because warrior diet is not basically an easy diet. You will need to mould your body slowly into following this particular eating pattern. There are benefits as well as disadvantages. I will cover all of them one by one. The most of the problems especially for women occur when they go into eating binge cycle after a long day of starvation. I will also recommend contacting your health professional before embarking on this journey. Many of the successful intermittent fasting articles are often written by young ripped men. Women have very different physiology. Occasionally, a fast once in a while is quite safe and healthy. However, if you want to make it your lifestyle as a woman, you must make sure it never messes up with your hormones or energy levels.

CHAPTER 6
FOOD TO EAT DURING INTERMITTENT FASTING FOR WOMEN OVER 50

We will look at some of the foods that you simply must include in your diet while you take up the fast.

Water

This is definitely the most important element to consume when you take up the intermittent fast. Water can act as an elixir when it comes to losing weight. You must keep your body hydrated and ensure that all the toxins are dissolved and eliminated. All your organs need water to remain fresh and healthy; right from your liver to gut to digestive tract, water helps to keep these organs working smoothly. Drink at least 8 to 10 glasses of water a day and focus more on the fasting period. It is obvious that it will get a little monotonous and so, a good idea is to consume fruit infused water. This refers to water that has fruit and herbs infused into it. Fill up a jar with water and toss in fruit and herbs such as oranges, lemons, mint leaves and a dash of cinnamon. Consume this every few hours. Remember that the intermittent fast can be quite taxing at times and lead to side effects such as headache and nausea. In such a case, only water can help you out and put an end to these.

Fish

Fish can be considered as a miracle food as it can greatly help with weight loss. According to dietary guidelines, it is important for people to consume at least 6 to 8 ounces of fish every week. Fish contains a lot of nutrients. It is rich in fats and proteins. It is also rich in vitamin D. and this means you do not have to worry about denying your body these nutrients by taking on the fast. You do not have to reach for supplements if you are able to consume fish regularly. Fish is also rich in DHA, which helps in brain development. You will see that your mind is fresher and you are able to think well. Your productivity will increase and stress will be curbed.

Avocado

You might wonder why avocado is in this list considering it is one of the fattiest foods out there. However, you must understand that the fasting phase can take a toll on your body and so you must consume foods that can keep you going. Avocado is rich in monounsaturated fat, which is great for those who tend to get hungry quite fast. It keeps you feeling full for longer. You will not find yourself reaching out to eat a snack. Avocado is quite versatile and can be added to your breakfast or lunch menu. Those who tend to include it in their breakfast menu are generally able to go without food for longer periods of time without complaining about hunger.

Leafy greens

If there is one type of vegetable that we remember being told to consume by our parents then it has to be leafy green vegetables. As we know, leafy green vegetables are loaded with multiple nutrients that are great for your body. These include the likes of kale, broccoli, lettuce, etc. These are loaded with fiber. Fiber, as you know, keeps your body going when you suffer from digestive issues such as constipation. You are sure to go through it when you adopt the intermittent fast. In such a case, it becomes that much more important to consume these vegetables to keep your stomach in good shape. Fiber also makes you feel fuller and not feel too hungry between meals.

Potatoes

As mentioned earlier, the goal is to consume foods that are filling and can keep you going for hours, one such being potatoes. Potatoes are rich in carbs that can keep you sated for hours. Make sure you either steam and mash them or roast them without the addition of any oil or fat. Deep frying them is never an option. Try to consume them with their skin on as the skin contains a lot of nutrition.

Probiotics

When it comes to digestion, both your liver and gut play a very important role. Both of them need a healthy dose of probiotics in order to function optimally. If you have an unhealthy gut then you might suffer from side effects such as constipation and even leaky gut syndrome. The best way to combat these is by consuming as many probiotics as possible. Some natural foods rich in probiotics include kombucha and kefir. Add these to your meals and you are sure to experience positive benefits. An alternative is to go for probiotic supplements. Make sure you know which ones to go for. It would be best to consult a physician first.

Assorted berries

There is nothing better than consuming fresh berries in the mornings. They are loaded with antioxidants and vital nutrients required to keep your body healthy. Strawberries, raspberries, blueberries and gooseberries all are great for you. Just toss them into the blender with some milk or yogurt to make a smoothie. According to studies, those who consumed berries regularly were able to remain within their ideal body weight and did not gain too much weight over longer periods of time.

Eggs

An important aspect of losing weight is building lean muscles. Lean muscles replace regular ones and prevent fat from getting stored. The best way to build lean muscle is by consuming foods rich in proteins. One important source of proteins is eggs. Those who consume eggs for breakfast are in a better position to develop lean muscles and not go hungry before the next meal. Eggs can be quite versatile and cooked in any way you like. Hard-boil them the previous day so that you have a ready meal the next morning. Simply toss them in a pan to scramble them. It only takes a few minutes to cook them.

Whole grains

One aspect of maintaining a clean and healthy diet is going for whole grains. The intermittent fast promotes consumption of these, as they are easier for the body to digest and keep the system clean. They are also loaded with proteins and fiber. Do not limit yourself to the usual such as wheat and oats and go for something different such as Bulgar, amaranth and flax.

Legumes

If you wish to remain full for longer and not feel hungry or peckish too often then there is nothing better than legumes and beans. These cannot only be quite flavorful but also loaded with fiber. The body does not easily digest fiber. In fact, the body cannot digest it at all but makes extra effort in trying to digest it thereby drawing into the fat reserves. It is, therefore, best to load up on fiber in order to lose weight easily. There are many options to pick from including peas, lentils, green beans, fava, black-eyed peas, etc. These easily fit into soups and salads.

Nuts

Nuts are fatty no doubt, but they contain good fat. Not all fat is bad fat as there can be some good fat as well. Polyunsaturated fats are said to be good for the body and can keep you feeling full for longer. You will not feel hungry if you munch on some walnuts or almonds. But make sure you make them a part of your meal and do not snack on them. Snacking on them can leave you feeling full and disrupt your meal plan. Do not worry about the calorie aspect. Nuts are not as calorific as you may have thought. They contain far less calories than some of the other fatty foods that people tend to snack on.

These happen to be superfoods that you must include in your diet while you take up intermittent fasting.

Foods to Avoid While Intermittent Fasting

Processed foods

Processed foods include the likes of biscuits, wafers, chips, cakes and sugary drinks such as cola. These will only add to your woes and counteract your weight loss goals. Try to avoid these at all costs. Do not hit the aisles at the supermarket that carry these foods. Remember to never go shopping on an empty stomach, as you will feel tempted to reach for a packet or snack.

Junk foods

Make it a point to cut out all junk food from your diet. There should be no room for burgers, pizzas and pastas that contain a lot of fat. It might be tempting to go for a cheat meal once in a while, but it is important not to do so as it can lead to a habit.

Alcohol

Although wine is said to be quite healthy, it would be best to limit it to just 1 serving per week. Try your best to avoid consuming hard liquor.

Although it is said that the intermittent fast does not tell you what not to eat, it is best to avoid these when you wish to lose weight.

With intermittent fasting, a lot of people tend to follow their usual eating habits in terms of the specific foods that they put on their plate during each meal, expecting that they will lose weight just because they have fasted during the morning, night, and a part of the afternoon.

While intermittent fasting may help to improve metabolism and support digestive function that will ultimately improve your ability to lose weight, the food you eat still counts. As you might have noted, the meal plans that I shared with you in this cookbook generally combines a range of healthy foods in order to ensure you get the nutrients you need without loading up on too many carbs. I did include a lot of delicious options that you can try out.

Just as there are a lot of foods that you can surely include in your diet to help you lose that extra weight that is causing you concern, there are also some foods that you should always try to avoid if your goal is to lose weight.

Below, I would like to share some of the most important foods that you should try to exclude from your diet in order to improve the results you are able to achieve when you implement the recipes and meal plans I have provided you within this book.

• Fried foods, of course, should be at the top of my list. There is no doubt that fried foods are one particularly common reason for the world to be so obese. Millions of people eat fried foods as much as every day. This does not only cause them to gain in weight, but also to experience a rise in cholesterol levels, be at a higher risk of heart disease, and more.

•	Fast foods, along with fried foods, since most chains that offer fast foods tend to deep fry their food in the worst types of oil and fat to make them more 'tasty' for the general public. Unfortunately, this also adds more fat to your belly, thighs, arms, and other areas of your body.

•	Corn is another food that really isn't the best choice for people who are trying to lose weight. Sure, it is not an unhealthy food, but consider the fact that this is a type of grain that is relatively high in sugar. The sugar spike experienced when you eat corn leads to the release of insulin, triggering inflammation and taking you one step closer to the dreadful complications of insulin resistance.

In addition to all of these, be sure to be wary of added sugars in everything you eat. For example, if you visit your local supermarket and grab a healthy bar to use as the food to break your fast, the fact that the word "healthy" appears on the bar does not necessarily mean it is truly healthy.

Always look at the ingredients of what you buy and what you will be putting into your body. Making your own healthy energy bars at home might be a better solution as well.

CHAPTER 7
INTERMITTENT FASTING 16/8 PLAN FOR WOMEN OVER 50

The 16/8 is a method of fasting done to achieve good health or even lose weight. You have to spend sixteen hours without taking any food; surviving on sugarless drinks such as herbal tea or mineral water. The other eight hours are left open and free for you to eat any meal of your choice. Within these eight hours, you are unrestricted to any specific foods. Intermittent fasting dates back to the time of our ancestors, who could hunt or gather during the day, eat, sleep, and do their fasting during the night. It is all equal to the 16/8 method of intermittent fasting.

There are no regulations on which meals you should skip, but the scientists have ascertained that skipping breakfast is okay as no facts that show that breakfast makes you more or less healthier.

Once you have consulted your physician and they recommend the 16/8 for you or tell you that you are fit for this kind of fasting, then you are good to go. It would be an added advantage practicing the 16/8 method if you have tried fasting before, but if you are doing it for the first time, then you need to do it gradually.

You can gradually increase your fasting hours from the 5/2 to 12-hour diet plan, then add a little more hour up to 16 hours then you are good to go. But then again, you should always listen to your body's response to these types of fasting and note the changes.

If you have tried fasting before, your body must have adjusted to energy changes and steaming this method of intermittent fasting with light exercises, and sugarless drinks keep your body fit. It should not be a point of concern if you find it hard to exercise during fasting periods; it is all normal and okay since human beings bodies are not the same. It is a method since after fasting, it gives you enough freedom to consume what you feel like eating, but it should not be an excuse to overeat junk foods. It is strictly clean and healthy meals.

You should avoid highly processed foods during non-fasting times. The following is an example, if not a hint of what you should try eating during the eight-hour non-fasting period:

Early consumption space

8 a.m. – you can take eggs and vegetable scrambles.

Noon – you take apples and almond butter.

Evening – you take chicken and vegetable stir.

If it is midday consumption space, start your day by taking a cup of black tea in the morning.

At 11 a.m., you may banana smoothies.

At 2 p.m. – take avocado toasted bread.

At 4 p.m. – take dark chocolate.

At 6 p.m. – take chicken meatballs with tomato sauce.

If you opt for late consumption window, drink a cup of black coffee before noon.

At 1 p.m. – take blackberry chia dessert.

At 4 p.m. – take carrots and guacamole.

Then at 9 p.m. – take grilled salmon with veggies.

You can make your meals appear simple but at the same time very healthy. You do not have to restrict yourself to taking five hundred calories, but provided you eat healthy and clean meals within the non-fasting eight hours; you will still achieve your goals. With this method of fasting, you will not be like you would do if you opted for the 5/2 diet plan.

The 16/8 is getting popular, even the world's famous personalities and celebrities are practicing this type of intermittent fasting.

CHAPTER 8

BEST EXERCISE TO LOSE WEIGHT AFTER 50 YEARS OLD

At 50, the topic of losing weight and fitness comes to the fore. As estrogen levels drop, the risk of accumulating pounds increases. By reducing the production of sex hormones during menopause, the body's energy requirements decrease and the basal metabolism decreases.

The growth hormone somatotropin, which helps build muscle, is also released less and less. This factor is associated with problems such as changes in body composition, muscle mass is lost, fat tissue builds up from 40 years of age. The metabolism slows down, which also reduces the calorie requirement.

From the age of 50, an almost daily, but shorter workout is recommended to lose weight. Joint-friendly sports such as aqua fitness, swimming or cycling are suitable for boarding. You can also start with 50 new sports: gentle yoga, tai chi, Nordic walking or even climbing. Since the age of 50 there is a risk of redistribution of body fat (more belly fat, less rounding on the hips and buttocks), targeted training on equipment is recommended to build muscle where fat is to be distributed. It is best to have special exercises shown during an introductory training session in the gym.

To keep your weight down, make it easy for yourself and

incorporate more exercise into your everyday life. Think about what habits you can change. The classic: climbing stairs instead of an elevator. If your joints and back allow it, you should do your shopping on foot: carrying half an hour of bags consumes around 140 calories. If you don't want to drag, take the bike. Car and bus should be off limits for shorter distances anyway. Gardening is also a good program against flab. Raking half an hour of leaves burns about 160 calories. Or complete a moderate exercise program with walking or walking every day.

Fitness exercise suitable for women over 50

Depending on your physical condition, all types of jogging, walking, swimming, cycling or hiking are highly recommended as endurance sports. Healthy training for the cardiovascular system can, of course, also be done easily indoors, for example on the cross trainer or rowing machine, in special fitness courses or online at home.

During endurance sports, high stress peaks due to possible cardiovascular diseases are to be avoided urgently. In cases of doubt, it is advisable to exercise with a heart rate monitor in order to remain in the optimal, healthy heart rate range.

Small devices such as Thera bands are very suitable for strength training, they offer optimal safety for the joints and can also be used wonderfully at home or on the go.

In addition to endurance and strength training, it is also important to train the coordination and the associated control of the proprioceptors in the body. Position, sense of movement, strength and balance can be trained and improved through targeted exercises. Exercises such as the one-legged stand serve, among other things, to prevent falls.

Incidentally, physical training also improves mental fitness through improved oxygen supply and the perceptual and cognitive challenge.

Four exercises to keep fit for women 50 years and above

Strengthen leg muscles

Stand next to a chair and hold on to the backrest. With the upper body upright and without kinking at the waist, raise the knee as far as possible towards the chest (if the hip is artificial, lift the thigh at most to the horizontal), slowly lower the leg again and repeat the exercise with the other leg.

Execution: Two series with ten repetitions per leg, always alternating between the left and right leg (so count to 20). In order to intensify the exercise, weight cuffs can also be put on above the ankles; a kilo is enough to start with.

Strengthen hips

Stand behind a chair and hold on to the backrest. Move one leg straight to the side without bending your waist or knees. The toes point forward during the movement. Slowly move the leg back to the starting position and repeat the exercise with the other leg.

Execution: Two series with ten repetitions per leg, always

alternating between the left and right leg (count to 20). To increase the effect, weight cuffs can also be put on above the ankles.

Strong upper arms

Sit upright on the front half of the chair surface. Grip the armrests of the chair so that your hands are right next to your torso. Put your feet forward. If possible, push your body up with your arms only, stretching your elbows as far as possible. Slowly sink back into the chair, trying to slow the movement with your arms. Take a deep breath and repeat the exercise.

Execution: Two series with ten repetitions each (with both arms at the same time).

For feet and calf muscles

Stand upright behind a chair and hold on to the backrest. Push your heels off the floor so that you stand on tiptoe. Slowly return to the starting position until the feet are firmly on the floor. Then lift both toes of your feet so that you stand on your heels.

Execution: two to three series with ten to 20 repetitions on both legs or ten repetitions each with one leg. Tip: Gradually increase up to 20 reps. If you find this too easy, try to lift your body weight only on the right or left leg.

CHAPTER 9
BEST RECIPES

Coated Cauliflower Head

Preparation time: 10 minutes

Cooking time: 40 minutes

Servings:6

Ingredients:

- 2-pound cauliflower head

- 3 tablespoons olive oil

- 1 tablespoon butter, softened

- 1 teaspoon ground coriander

- 1 teaspoon salt

- 1 egg, whisked

- 1 teaspoon dried cilantro

- 1 teaspoon dried oregano

- 1 teaspoon tahini paste

Directions:

1. Trim cauliflower head if needed.

2. Preheat oven to 350F.

3. In the mixing bowl, mix up together olive oil, softened butter, ground coriander, salt, whisked egg, dried cilantro, dried oregano, and tahini paste.

4. Then brush the cauliflower head with this mixture generously and transfer in the tray.

5. Bake the cauliflower head for 40 minutes.

6. Brush it with the remaining oil mixture every 10 minutes.

Nutrition: calories 131, fat 10.3, fiber 4, carbs 8.4, protein 4.1

Artichoke Petals Bites

Preparation time: 10 minutes

Cooking time: 10 minutes

Servings:8

Ingredients:

- 8 oz artichoke petals, boiled, drained, without salt

- ½ cup almond flour

- 4 oz Parmesan, grated

- 2 tablespoons almond butter, melted

Directions:

1. In the mixing bowl, mix up together almond flour and grated Parmesan.

2. Preheat the oven to 355F.

3. Dip the artichoke petals in the almond butter and then coat in the almond flour mixture.

4. Place them in the tray.

5. Transfer the tray in the preheated oven and cook the petals for 10 minutes.

6. Chill the cooked petal bites little before serving.

Nutrition: calories 140, fat 6.4, fiber 7.6, carbs 14.6, protein 10

Stuffed Beef Loin in Sticky Sauce

Preparation time: 15 minutes

Cooking time: 6 minutes

Servings:4

Ingredients:

- 1 tablespoon Erythritol
- 1 tablespoon lemon juice
- 4 tablespoons water
- 1 tablespoon butter
- ½ teaspoon tomato sauce
- ¼ teaspoon dried rosemary
- 9 oz beef loin
- 3 oz celery root, grated
- 3 oz bacon, sliced

- 1 tablespoon walnuts, chopped

- ¾ teaspoon garlic, diced

- 2 teaspoons butter

- 1 tablespoon olive oil

- 1 teaspoon salt

- ½ cup of water

Directions:

1. Cut the beef loin into the layer and spread it with the dried rosemary, butter, and salt.

2. Then place over the beef loin: grated celery root, sliced bacon, walnuts, and diced garlic.

3. Roll the beef loin and brush it with olive oil.

4. Secure the meat with the help of the toothpicks.

5. Place it in the tray and add a ½ cup of water.

6. Cook the meat in the preheated to 365F oven for 40 minutes.

7. Meanwhile, make the sticky sauce: mix up together Erythritol, lemon juice, 4 tablespoons of water, and butter.

8. Preheat the mixture until it starts to boil.

9. Then add tomato sauce and whisk it well.

10. Bring the sauce to boil and remove from the heat.

11. When the beef loin is cooked, remove it from the oven and brush with the cooked sticky sauce very generously.

12. Slice the beef roll and sprinkle with the remaining sauce.

Nutrition: calories 248, fat 17.5, fiber 0.5, carbs 2.2, protein 20.7

BBQ Pork Tenders

Preparation time: 15 minutes

Cooking time: 7 minutes

Servings:4

Ingredients:

- 1 teaspoon Erythritol
- 3 tablespoons ground paprika
- 1 teaspoon ground black pepper
- 1 teaspoon salt
- ½ teaspoon chili powder
- ¼ teaspoon cayenne pepper
- 1 teaspoon garlic powder
- 14 oz pork loins
- 1 tablespoon olive oil
- 1 tablespoon almond butter

Directions:

1. Make the BBQ mix: in the shallow bowl, mix up together ground paprika, Erythritol, ground black pepper, salt, chili powder, cayenne pepper, garlic powder.

2. Cut the pork loin into the tenders.

3. Rub every pork loin with BBQ mix and sprinkle with olive oil.

4. Leave the meat to marinate for at least 15 minutes.

5. After this, place almond butter in the skillet and melt it.

6. Place the pork tenders in the almond butter and cook them for 5 minutes.

7. Then flip the meat onto another side and cook for 2 minutes more. The time of cooking depends on meat thickness.

Nutrition: calories 315, fat 20.3, fiber 2.7, carbs 4.7, protein 29

Fish Bars

Preparation time: 10 minutes

Cooking time: 15 minutes

Servings:6

Ingredients:

- 10 oz tilapia fillet

- ½ cup coconut flour

- 2 eggs, whisked

- 1 teaspoon salt

- ½ teaspoon ground black pepper

- 3 oz Parmesan, grated

- 1 teaspoon butter

Directions:

1. Mince the tilapia fillet and place it in the mixing bowl.

2. Add coconut flour, whisked eggs, salt, ground black pepper, and grated cheese.

3. Mix up the mixture with the help of the spoon until homogenous.

4. Spread the casserole mold with the butter generously.

5. Place the fish mixture in the mold and flatten it well. Cut the mixture into the bars with the help of the knife.

6. Preheat the oven to 360F.

7. Place the casserole mold in the oven and cook the fish bars for 15 minutes or until the fish bars get the golden-brown surface.

8. Chill the cooked meal well and only after this, transfer it in the serving plates.

Nutrition: calories 128, fat 5.8, fiber 0.5, carbs 1.4, protein 17.6

Pan-fried Cod

Preparation time: 5 minutes

Cooking time: 10 minutes

Servings:2

Ingredients:

- 12 oz cod fillet

- 1 tablespoon scallions, chopped

- 1 tablespoon butter

- 1 tablespoon coconut oil

- 1 teaspoon garlic, diced

- 1 teaspoon cumin seeds

- 1 teaspoon coriander seeds

- 1 teaspoon salt

Directions:

1. Place butter and coconut oil in the skillet and melt them.

2. Add garlic, cumin and coriander seeds.

3. Rub the fish fillet with salt and place it in the skillet.

4. Fry the fish for 2 minutes from each side or until it is light brown.

5. Transfer the cooked cod fillet in the plate and cut into 2 servings.

6. Nutrition: calories 253, fat 14.3, fiber 0.2, carbs 1.2,
    protein 30.8

82

CHAPTER 10
MOST COMMON MISTAKES TO AVOID

Intermittent fasting is an eating pattern, not a diet pattern. Some people usually get it wrong. I have already given a subsection before, telling you every detail about the intermittent fasting and how to get it right. As a woman above fifty, there is a lot that needs to be taken care of in your body. Women above fifty have a very different body than young females and most certainly men. The females have a lot of processes and hormonal phases that are very different than men. For females above fifty, the processes are even different than younger females. Therefore, there are a number of mistakes often done by women above fifty which can harm their health.

There is a reason why I have constantly asked you, considering you are a woman above fifty, to go and check your health plan with a proper nutritionist. Women have a sensitive health and their bodies in general are more sensitive to intermittent fasting. However, here is something to consider. As a younger female, your body is quite flexible. It can heal and deal with the issues which the body of an aged female cannot. Therefore, as a younger female, you can experiment with your body more often and still recoil if a harmful effect occurs. For example, some women in twenties experience stomach issues and acidity due to fasting. They can still become quite active after dropping intermittent fasting. Chances are, a young female will easily be able to recoil after a health issue in a matter of days. For aged women, this is really not the case. Your body needs care since it is weaker than when you were in your thirties or even forties. Your body will need proper care. That is one of the reasons why before trying out any new method, you need to consult a health professional. If your body experiences harmful effects from the method of intermittent fasting, it may take more days and sometimes even a week or two to properly recover. I know I have explained it time to time that you should experiment with what works best. However, this is one of the mistakes made by women above fifty. I will gently explain how you should be experimenting with your fifty years old body. The main purpose is really to adopt a system of health that works best for you. That system shouldn't really impede your health or shouldn't really do opposite of what you were trying to achieve. Secondly, you should be gentle with your body. In a way, I am saying that as an aged woman, you should do controlled experiment with your body in trying to find out what works and what doesn't. I would really recommend discussing those methods with a health professional or at least checking online to see if what you are doing is suitable for you or not. Given below are the most common mistakes made by women above fifty that can be harmful during intermittent fasting.

1. Combining Intermittent Fasting with a nutrient deficient dieting pattern:

I have recently been studying a book about ketogenic diet. Some nutritionists have combined it with the intermittent fasting for successful results. People have done this and recorded successful results. Ketogenic diet is basically a diet pattern in which you are feeding your body very low carbs and high amount of fats. This makes the body enter into the state of ketosis that can easily burn more fats and reduce weight. However, this approach alone is harmful for the people near age fifty.

If you combine intermittent fasting with a dieting pattern without getting a medical advice, then that will be counter to your health. I cannot emphasize enough how this one mistake can cost you. There are multiple reasons for that. The first reason is that females have a very different body. Their bodies respond differently to some nutrition deficiency than men. Keto diet generally proved most effective for most people. However, it didn't do much to provide benefits for everyone. Among the ones it doesn't benefit are the people above fifty or people near that age.

As a woman above fifty, your body is now producing those proteins in smaller amount than before. Intermittent fasting alone is enough stress on a regular body. For people above fifty, it is already a big change. Combining it with a diet that restricts eating certain foods is not the smartest move. It is quite a big mistake made by females who are aged. Your body as a fifty years old woman needs those proteins and balanced meals. Every nutrient and protein that comes in your body is required for your body's growth and functions.

Furthermore, there are a few diets that can be very harmful to females facing menopause. Intermittent fasting alone is not recommended for females facing menopause. Consider what would happen when you combine it with a dieting pattern at such a phase. The result will be uncontrollable mood swings, heat flashes and many other adverse side effects that you will not foresee. Better take precautions and stick alone to intermittent fasting. At this age, it is beneficial for you alone.

2.   Suddenly Changing it all:

This would not be a smart move especially for a female your age. I have explained earlier that as an aged woman, your body is slow in making changes. Your body is quite slow in producing proteins and nutrients that you need.

Some aged females make the mistake of trying prolonged fasting as beginners. They suddenly jump into action, aiming straight for the twenty-four hours fast plan. Alternatively, many females take a start with 16/8 diet. While that is wonderful, make sure you are not over exerting yourself. Some aged women fall into the much-abused hype of skipping breakfast and going straight for the lunch. I cannot emphasize enough how this is a wrong approach.

If you are an aged woman who has never skipped breakfast, I wouldn't recommend trying it now in the name of intermittent fasting. Similarly, if you have never made sudden changes in your life like that of intermittent fasting, I wouldn't recommend making them now.

Make changes that will be comfortable with your body. If you have to skip a meal, I would recommend starting out with breakfast if you take it regularly. Make sure to take in proper and balanced meal. Then, you can start your day. I would advise delaying the regular lunch time by an hour or two. Your body can actually take it. You will then be having a proper lunch and then onwards, you will be having the fast. This approach is recommended for the females above fifty since it is quite suitable for you. You are not skipping any breakfast. You are simply going on with your normal routine, only modified it a little bit. If you start your day without breakfast, then by all means take a healthy lunch and pass your day. At night, stack yourself with a healthy dinner and then you will be ready. The benefit with this approach is that you will be spending eight to nine hours in sleeping. This will make your fast pass easier. If you already have a routine then find a style of intermittent fasting that goes along with that routine.

Furthermore, make sure your body can take the change that you have already made. If you find yourself fairly comfortable with it, then move on to advanced methods. It is quite possible you start with a bigger window of eating and shorter window of fasting. That will work well too! As a woman above fifty, make change that suits you.

3.   Snacking Unhealthily during Fasting:

A particularly interesting way to cope up with the intermittent fasting is taking in liquids during the fasting window. It is recommended that you don't enter into starvation mode. You should take small snacks to pass your time and keep your body supported. However, some females take it as an opportunity to take in unhealthy snacks.

Some snacks such as chips from market or those small muffins you gobbled are not a good way to pass the fasting time. You are taking in unhealthy meals and you are making your body take in more unhealthy calories. You shouldn't really take in those things. I would recommend choosing a fasting window that is mostly passed in sleep and a little time of waiting. If you keep on eating unhealthy snacks during the fasting period and tell yourself you skipped a meal due to intermittent fasting, then it is not making a difference. As a woman above fifty, the unhealthy snacks are going to be even more harmful for your aged body than those of younger females. I would recommend eating vegetables or fruits. The best healthy snack that I would recommend is the berries. The berries are healthy fruits and eating handful of them is quite refreshing.

4.   Not enough Hydration:

The most critical point while doing the intermittent fasting is remaining hydrated. The lack of water can lead to some complications. Dehydration alone is quite an unhealthy state of body. Our body may respond differently for different cases.

However, in case of women above fifty, the dehydration can lead to some problems which are not common among young people. There is a reason for it. As a female above fifty, you will need to take care of the body. Some people make the mistake of treating the fasting window as something similar to a starvation period. You cannot do that!

Dehydration's first most obvious sign is that you will feel thirsty. However, as a fifty years old woman, you may not feel like that. Your body will react differently to the dehydration than simple thirst. Quite possibly, you may not even feel dehydrated.

For mild dehydration, you would feel something like dry mouth sticky mouth. Furthermore, the lack of proper water can also lead to sleeplessness or fatigue in general. Headaches and light headedness is also possible. As an aged woman, you will need to stay hydrated. You can see that simple thirst is not an obvious sign of dehydration at this age.

In case of severe dehydration, the symptoms become more severe. You can see for yourself that in some cases, you will notice very dry mouth. The conditions like extreme fatigue or even extreme confusion. Your mucous membranes are going to respond abnormally. The heart beat is going to be faster than usual. You may contact high fever and in extreme cases, there may be very low energy, leading to unconsciousness.

You will need to avoid being dehydrated at all costs. In fasting window, you can sip water or black tea or coffee without sweets.

The main reason why I prefer eating fruits or vegetables during snacking is because they contain enough water to avoid dehydration. Furthermore, I would also suggest doing proper analysis on how much water to drink. Normally, for people, you will have to drink 2 litres of water a day. This means you will be sipping in seven to eight glasses of water a day. Furthermore, look for the signs above. Don't ignore them as common weakness as most aged women do. It is quite normal to get weakness during fifties. However, if you are experiencing these symptoms especially if you are fasting, consider the possibility of dehydration.

Best case scenario would be talking to your doctor and finding out how much you really need. If your body requires lesser water, than keep in mind to drink that much. It is fairly common for aged women to require lesser amount of water than needed for younger females.

5.   Eating Unhealthy Foods during Eating Window:

Some women above fifty make the biggest mistake of eating unhealthy foods during intermittent fasting. Some of these foods are not suitable for people over fifty. Since women around this age also fall into this category, you will need to avoid certain foods too. I will give a list of all of them.

Many women above fifty make the mistake of eating foods which their doctors have advised against. They use intermittent fasting as an excuse since it is a healthy eating pattern. Just because intermittent fasting doesn't restrict what to eat and what to avoid, doesn't mean you should eat foods that are unhealthy. The reason why some foods are not allowed for you are is just extra calories. The extra calories will definitely be cut down when you start with intermittent fasting. However, some of these foods are not suitable for you as a woman above fifty. Some of these can easily raise your blood pressure that can be harmful for aged people. Similarly, some foods are going to cause more harm than good. Why? When you are doing intermittent fasting, what you eat later in eating is all you will be eating. Now imagine if you only eat those unhealthy foods that your doctor specifically advised against eating. Your body will have reactions that you will not like. Your body will simply reject those foods. Make sure you don't binge on unhealthy foods. Given below is the list of foods that may prove very harmful for you. These foods are given below. Make sure you aren't eating them in your regular eating window.

1. Avoid eating pickles at this age. The pickle is not suited for aged women for many reasons. But how? Doesn't eating vegetables actually improve your health? Well, not processed vegetables. The chief reason behind the pickles being excluded out of eating list is because pickles contain sodium. The sodium is a food that naturally increases your blood pressure. As a woman above fifty, your blood pressure is the top priority of your health. You will need to cut down on foods that increase your blood pressure and the pickles are one of them. All of the foods that have more than appropriate amount of salt fall into this category.

2.   Processed potatoes are a big no. Why? Potatoes contain starch that you will need to keep under control. If potatoes are cut into fries or sprinkled with bacons. Potatoes are generally healthy but only if they are not sprinkled with extras that have many harmful ingredients in them. Make sure to eat potatoes are bare without extras as possible. Boiled potatoes are good.

3.   Pastries are a big no. Why? The cream that is used in them along with extra sweets that can easily throw your blood pressure off balance. As women around this age, you will need to watch your sugar levels. Having sugar levels above the normal ones will not just cause hyperactivity but hyper blood pressure too. Cut down on pastries and don't even think of starting your breakfast from them.

4.   Butter is another big no. The saturated fats will easily increase your cholesterol and your chances of heart diseases. I would recommend swapping butter with olive oil or nuts.

5.   Red wine is generally good for you as long as you keep in under moderation. However, drinking too much wine is quite harmful. You will need to keep yourself from sipping extra glasses of wine. There are a lot of other ingredients within wine that will prove to be quite harmful for you.

6.   Deli meat sandwiches are an easy meal that are easily available and are often a great substitute for regular meals. However, the deli meats are not going to be a healthy choice once you cross your fifties. Instead of deli meats, please go for the lean meats in

your sandwiches. They are going to be far healthier than your deli meat sandwich or deli meat meal.

7.   Steam bag frozen vegetables are another kind of foods that many women mistake for regular vegetables. The steamed bag frozen vegetables are creams, sauces and salts that are not going to be good for you. Some steamed vegetables are full of salts and sauces that may raise your blood pressure.

8.   Deep dish pizza is another unhealthy food that is taken as a healthy one. No one actually cares that salty topping with a heavy amount of cheese is unhealthy for most of the people. Eating it in small amounts as a snack is not a bad idea. However, for females around fifty, making it a diet is something seriously harmful. Please consider this next time when you eat pizza as a way of breaking your fast.

9.   Bacon is another one of the foods that is high in salt and ingredients. It will increase your blood pressure to unhealthy levels and that is something quite troublesome. You can eat it at sometimes but not on regular basis.

10. Cherries are packed with sugar. Balance the diet with proper nutrients. If you keep on eating cherries on every meal, they are not going to be healthy. Generally, eating everything in excess amount is going to be unhealthy. However, cherries are the fruits you will need to avoid more. Eating it sometimes is favourable.

11. Chicken skin is another food that you will have to avoid in this age. The chicken baked as a whole is quite a healthy dish.

However, eating it with skin is not recommended. It is another one of the foods that you will need to avoid once you cross fifty.

12. Soda drinks are a big no. The soda drinks have plenty of sugar and they will easily raise diabetes risk. Even for younger people, too many soda drinks can lead to poor health. The women above fifty should avoid it at all costs.

13. Grapes are another type of fruits that you should eat in low quantities. Their high carb and high sugar can make it difficult.

6.   Overeating after the breaking of Fast:

The overeating is also a disorder known as binge eating disorder. According to a research, above 30 million Americans have this disorder. Among those Americans, thirteen percent are older women above fifty. It is quite an interesting fact that we only picture teenagers or middle aged people with overeating disorder. However, it is also something found in elder women. Even if you had not developed the overeating or binge-eating before, you may have developed it now. How?

Many women make the mistake of entering into the starvation state. They make the mistake of ignoring those sharp hunger pangs during fasting window of intermittent fasting. However, when the fasting window ends, they will end up binging on foods. Even when you are consuming the healthy foods and the diet consists of wheat and rice, the habit itself is quite unhealthy. This is the reason why we hear about some people gaining weight after fasting. This may actually be truer for the women above fifty. As an aged woman, you will need to keep your calories in check along with the rest of the diet. You will need to check if the calorie intake is more or lesser than what you are taking on everyday basis. In some cases, binge eating is also triggered by some traumatic events and sudden life transitions. I have personally read about multiple reports about females undergoing different difficult scenarios in which they had to resort to binge eating to cope up. If this is your situation, then you already had developed binge eating disorder. You can then seek therapy or consult your doctor for life changing and helpful transitions. However, in case if you developed binge eating disorder only because of intermittent fasting, the reason might be hidden in not listening to your body.

CHAPTER 11
INTERMITTENT FASTING TIPS AND TRICKS

P ractice indeed makes perfect. To help you get in the intermittent fasting, I have outlined a few down-to-earth routes and hands-on tips to guide you. Your approach to fasting can mean the difference between success and failure. So, consider these tips as guidelines that will help safely implement your preferred fasting regimen.

Find a Worthy Goal

First things first: find a goal that is worth pursuing, or else you will drop the idea at the first sign of resistance. If you don't have a goal that represents a strong ideal, it won't be long before you start telling yourself, "I think I've passed the stage of such childishness." And yes, many women start a new lifestyle change for reasons that they can't keep up when things get tough. For example, the desire to look like models on TV, or social media makes losing weight feel socially acceptable, and ok to keep up with trends that can be harmful. These reasons are not enough to keep anyone committed to a full lifestyle change and few wonder why so many people with goals are quick to jump from one lifestyle to another.

Don't go into fasting intermittently because it is the thing to do at the moment. Instead, look for inspiring goals such as:

96

- Staying fit, young, and healthy.

- Improving your cognitive or brain functions.

- Improving your overall vitality and increase energy levels.

- Balancing hormones, especially during menopausal or post-menopausal stages of life.

- Improving your overall health, thereby increasing longevity.

Do any of these sound good to you? Surely at this stage of your life, you are aware of the inherent risks of doing something merely because others are doing it too. That type of motivation will fail you.

Check Your Hormones

A woman's hormones can be easily thrown out of whack by the slightest change in her already established pattern of behavior. Whether it is a physical change such as altering your eating pattern or an emotional change such as being irritated or sad, it can bring about hormonal imbalance in a woman even if it is temporary.

But for the perimenopausal and menopausal women, hormones can go haywire for reasons even they can't define. She could be feeling really great all week, and without anything changing she could suddenly become fatigued, depressed, and not in the right frame of mind. These changes happen due to the unpredictability of this phase of a woman's life. Because this can happen for no apparent reason, it is best to check your hormonal levels before putting your body through a major lifestyle change. If you've ever had issues with thyroid, cortisol, or adrenal fatigue, ensure that you have these checks before you begin.

This may come as a surprise to some women, but your ovaries produce testosterone too. So, as you grow older and begin to experience a decline in your estrogen and progesterone levels, your testosterone levels are also taking a nosedive. Your libido can be affected by low levels of testosterone and make you feel exhausted and bummed-out for no reason at all. So while you are checking your other hormones, don't forget to do a testosterone test. The thyroid and testosterone hormones also help in weight regulation. So, if you intend to shed some weight using intermittent fasting, these tests are very necessary.

Start Slow

To go from having five or six meals daily to eating only once a day can lead to very dire consequences. In addition to being harmful to your health, massive abrupt changes are hardly sustainable. After confirming that intermittent fasting is suitable for your health, the next thing to do is planning how to ease into the habit. Take another look at the example of how to ease into fasting and consider following the example or coming up with something similar that works for you. In other words, before you fully implement any intermittent fasting regimen, it is a good practice to first test the waters, so to speak, with a less strict form of fasting. By doing this, it will help your body acclimate to the changes before going into the proper regimen.

Don't Fuss Over What You Can Eat

One common mistake people make when fasting is obsessing over the fasting hours and what to eat when they are finally allowed. You don't have to worry about if you are fasting as long as someone else, the important thing is what's comfortable for you. Of course, if your fasting window is too small, you are not likely to see any result. Also, don't get too tied up in every little detail of intermittent fasting. For example, you don't have to become too worried because you missed a day. Remember that fasting intermittently should be a lifestyle change if you want to continue to reap the benefits. And for a lifestyle change to be sustainable, you must be able to adapt and use it in a way that even if you face challenges, you will work your way around it somehow. Missing a day or cutting your fast short for reasons beyond your control shouldn't get you worked up and worrying about whether you can do the entire plan. Don't give up.

Again, some people focus too much on what they can eat or not eat. For example, "Can I add just a little butter or cream?" " Would it hurt to eat this type of food during the fasting window?" If your focus is on what you can have or eat while you are fasting, you are giving your attention to the wrong things and putting your mind in an unhelpful state. Give your mind the right focus by concentrating on doing a good, clean, fast, and try to consume only water, tea, or coffee during the window.

Watch Electrolytes

Your body electrolytes are compounds and elements that occur naturally in body fluids, blood, and urine. They can also be ingested through drinks, foods, and supplements. Some of them include magnesium, calcium, potassium, chloride, phosphate, and sodium. Their functions include fluid balance, regulation of the heart and neurological function, acid-base balance, oxygen delivery, and many other functions.

It is important to keep these electrolytes in a state of balance. But many people who practice fasting tend to neglect this and run into problems. Here is a common notion: "Don't let anything into your stomach until the end of your fast" Even those just starting to fast know it doesn't work that way, and they tend to forget or fully stay away from liquids during their fasting window.

When you lose too much water from your body through sweating, vomiting, and diarrhea, or you don't have enough water in your body because you don't drink enough liquids, you increase the risk of electrolyte disorders. It is not okay to drink tea or black coffee throughout the morning period of your fast window. You will wear yourself down if you don't drink enough water. The longer you fast without water, the higher your chances of flushing out electrolytes and running into trouble. You can end up raising your blood pressure, develop muscle twitching and spasms, fatigue, fast heart rate or irregular heartbeat, and many other health problems.

On the other hand, drinking too much water can also tip the water-electrolyte balance. What you want to do is to drink adequate amounts of water and not excess water, whether you are fasting or not.

Give the Calorie Restriction a Rest

Remember that intermittent fasting is different from dieting. Your focus should be on eating healthily during your eating window or eating days instead of focusing on calorie restriction. Even if you are fasting for weight loss, don't obsess over calories. Following a fasting regimen is enough to take care of the calories you consume. It is absolutely unnecessary to engage in a practice that can hurt your metabolism. Combining intermittent fasting with eating too little food in your eating window because you are worried about your calorie intake can cause problems for your metabolism.

One of the major reasons that people push themselves into restricting calories while fasting is their concern for rapid weight loss. You need to be wary of any process that brings about drastic physical changes to your body in very short amounts of time. While it is okay to desire quick results, your health and safety are more important. When you obsess or worry that you are not losing weight as quickly as you want, you are not helping matters. Instead, you are increasing your stress level, and that is counterproductive. You are already taking practical steps toward losing weight by intermittent fasting, why would you want to undo your hard work by unnecessary worrying?

Simply focus on following a sustainable intermittent fasting regimen and let go of the need to restrict your calorie intake. Intermittent fasting will give your body the right number of calories it needs if you do it properly.

The First Meal of the Eating Window Is Key

Breaking your fast is a crucial part of the process because if you don't get it right, it could quickly develop into unhealthy eating patterns. When you break your fast, it is important to have healthy foods around to prevent grabbing unhealthy feel good snacks. Make sure what you are eating in your window is not a high-sugar or high-carb meal. I recommend that you consider breaking your fast with something that is highly nutrient-dense such as a green smoothie, protein shake, or healthy salad.

As much as possible, avoid breaking your fast with foods from a fast-food restaurant. Eating junk foods after your fast is a quick way to ruin all the hard work you've put in during your fasting window. If, for any reason, you can't prepare your meal, ensure that you order very specific foods that will complement your effort and not destroy what you've built.

Break Your Fast Gently

It is okay to feel very hungry after going for a long time without food, even if you were drinking water all through the fasting window. This is particularly true for people who are just starting with fasting. But don't let the intensity of your hunger push you to eat. You don't want to force food hurriedly into your stomach after going long without food, or you might hurt yourself and experience stomach distress. Take it slow when you break your fast. Eat light meals in small portions first when you break your fast. Wait for a couple of minutes for your stomach to get used to the presence of food again before continuing with a normal-sized meal. The waiting period will douse any hunger pangs and remove the urge to rush your meal. For example, break your fast with a small serving of salad and wait for about 15 minutes. Drink some water and then after about five more minutes, you can eat a normal-sized meal.

Nutrition is Important

Although intermittent fasting is not dieting and so, does not specify which foods to eat, limit, and completely avoid, it makes sense to eat healthily. This means focusing on eating a balanced diet, such as:

1.   Whole grains

2.   Fruits and vegetables (canned in water, fresh, or frozen).

3.   Lean sources of protein (lentils, beans, eggs, poultry, tofu, and so on).

4.   Healthy fats (nuts, seeds, coconuts, avocados, olive oil, olive, and fatty fish).

It simply doesn't make any sense to go for 16 hours (or more) without food and then spend the rest of the day eating junk. Even if you follow the 5:2 diet and limit your calorie intake to only 500 calories per day for two days, it is totally illogical to follow it with five days of eating highly processed foods and low-quality meals. Combining intermittent fasting with unbalanced diets will lead to nutritional deficiencies and defeat the goal of fasting in the first place. Realize that intermittent fasting is not a magic wand that makes all poor eating habits vanish in a poof! For the practice to work, you must be deliberate about the types of food you eat.

Find a Regimen That Works for You

Don't follow a fasting diet because it seems to suit someone else. Instead, go for something that fits into your schedule. If you feel caged or boxed in by a particular fasting plan, it is a clear indication that it is not a suitable plan for you. Thankfully, you have the freedom to design something that works for you, even if you are following a specific regimen. The regimens are not carved in stone! They are flexible, and you can adjust them to suit you as long as you follow each regimen's basic principles. For example, if you decide to follow the 16:8 fasting regimen, your 8-hour eating window must not strictly be between noon and 8 pm. You have the option of tailoring the eating window to something that gives you room to handle other aspects of your life, such as work, hobbies, family, and so on. You might decide to make your 8-hour eating window from 9 am to 5 pm, or from 1 pm to 9 pm.

Whatever you choose to do is totally up to you. After all, it is your life, and you have the freedom to choose what you want. Books, the internet, and even loved ones can only suggest and offer recommendations. Ultimately, the final decision rests with you. Since your goal is not to please someone else or seek external approval, you should make your choice based on what is most convenient for you. You are seeking results, not accolades.

Therefore, don't follow something unrealistic for you or too restrictive. Even if you endure the most stringent type of fast and get admiration and commendation from others, have you considered what that fasting regimen is doing to your overall health? The female body is delicately designed, and putting it through unnecessary stress is unsafe if you are merely enduring discomfort to boost your ego.

Be Patient

Whatever propaganda you may have heard about fast results, the reality is that nothing is typical because we all have unique processes regardless of our physical appearance. Be patient even if others who began fasting at the same time are already seeing results and you have nothing to show for your efforts so far. It can be frustrating and discouraging but give your body time to adjust. As long as you don't have any medical reason to stop, don't give up just yet. Continue the practice for at least a month.

Realize that changes take time. There is no magic about the process of losing weight, improved vitality, or any other health benefits of intermittent fasting. Don't be in a hurry, and don't give people the room to put you under unnecessary pressure. Each person has their own pace, and it has absolutely nothing to do with you. If you continue to focus on other people's results or your seeming lack of results, you are giving your mind reasons to discontinue. Be patient.

CONCLUSION

Intermittent Fasting is a great option if you are desirous of burning body fat, lower weight, as well as developing better body shape. This diet plan is not only about the foods that you absorb. It is concerning the time of the day that you eat these foods to ensure that you can be well balanced and also healthy and balanced as well as additionally get your body to do the initiative for you.

The hardest part of this diet regimen is to instruct on your own to not consume at all times. We have been advised that we eat 5 or 6 meals a day (which is great if they're little dishes), yet this isn't the case for a lot of people. With Intermittent Fasting, you will be able to get the outcomes that you call for without needing to work so hard.

Low carbohydrate diet plans might suggest limiting carbs to 100 or perhaps 50 grams each day. This suggests cutting approach back on sugars, starches as well as all high carb foods. Obviously, this is far better for your body, because your pancreas does not require to work as tough to eliminate sugars from your system.

Intermittent fasting is not simply a weight-loss diet strategy. It means for more than that. It has a number of health and wellness benefits that will not just make you slimmer much healthier as well as disease-free. if you are taking into consideration reduced carbohydrate, Intermittent Fasting you will desire to see to it to review the entire message

Intermittent fasting recommends fasting for a figured out amount of time (whole lots of individuals quickly 24 hours after that consume healthy the next 24 hours, and more). This shows your body needs to scavenge around for food (fuel), as well as in the procedure does away with negative aged or broken cells and other waste that has created in your body.

It is essential to incorporate the two of these for "Low Carb Intermittent Fasting," and you are set to have a winning formula to help you attain weight reduction and a fantastic experience.

You should not eat foods for a 24 hour period when you are fasting you can still have reduced carb and reduced-calorie beverages such as water and also black coffee. You can eat healthily and balanced the adhering to day, but you must still maintain a watch on your carbohydrate intake. Examine out labels as well as research study foods to understand you are making the finest options for your body as well as your health and wellness.

This is a way of life modification and should be a constant technique of consuming for you (a minimum of the low carbs). You need to make a principles effort to make clever food as well as drink options!

Incorporate low carb intermittent fasting together with workout as well as you'll continue to be in shape before you recognize it and also will certainly feel fantastic.

Intermittent Fasting minimizes fat oxidation and also may decrease body weight. Exercising will certainly speed the process along and will certainly help you eliminate loose and flabby skin as well as get toned.

Intermittent fasting that has been performed on animals reveals a life-span increase of 40% or even more. That's amazing! This demonstrates exactly how much consuming healthy and balanced and also cleansing your body can benefit not just your system and also assist you lower weight, nevertheless, it can furthermore increase your days on this planet.

Reduced carbohydrate food choices are vegetables. You can fairly a lot consume as great deals of vegetables as you want. Meats and also fish are fantastic dinner choices. For lunch, you could make a salad with a boiled egg, onion and also a touch of cheese. See the carbs in the clothing nonetheless.

As long as you are recognized to make a healthy way of living selections, your need for carbohydrates and sugars will possibly be gone. That need will definitely be decreased! You'll no much longer want greasy, pleasant foods when you start choosing to consume healthy and balanced, low carb foods.

And also keep in mind prior to starting any kind of diet plan technique or workout routine, constantly talk to your health care specialist! You want to make sure you stay healthy and balanced while getting much healthier!

Many thanks for completing this book. I hope it was practical enough and able to provide you with the vital tools you need to attain your fitness goals.